KEY TOPICS IN

PLASTIC AND
RECONSTRUCTIVE SURGERY

The KEY TOPICS Series

Accident and Emergency Medicine, Second Edition
Anaesthesia: Clinical Aspects, Third Edition
Cardiac Surgery
Cardiovascular Medicine
Chronic Pain, Second Edition
Critical Care, Second Edition
Evidence-Based Medicine
Gastroenterology
General Surgery
Human Diseases for Dental Students
Neonatology, Second Edition
Neurology
Obstetrics and Gynaecology, Second Edition
Oncology
Ophthalmology, Second Edition
Oral and Maxillofacial Surgery
Orthopaedic Surgery
Orthopaedic Trauma Surgery
Otolaryngology, Second Edition
Paediatrics, Second Edition
Pain Management, Second Edition
Psychiatry
Renal Medicine
Respiratory Medicine
Sexual Health
Thoracic Surgery
Trauma

KEY TOPICS IN
PLASTIC AND RECONSTRUCTIVE SURGERY

Tor Wo Chiu
Assistant Professor of Plastic and Reconstructive Surgery
Department of Surgery
Prince of Wales Hospital
Shatin
Hong Kong SAR
China

Andrew Burd
Professor of Plastic and Reconstructive Surgery
Department of Surgery
Prince of Wales Hospital
Shatin
Hong Kong SAR
China

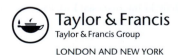
Taylor & Francis
Taylor & Francis Group

LONDON AND NEW YORK

© 2005 Taylor & Francis, an imprint of the Taylor & Francis Group
Taylor & Francis Group is the Academic Division of T&F Informa plc

First published in the United Kingdom in 2005
by Taylor & Francis, an imprint of the Taylor & Francis Group,
2 Park Square, Milton Park, Abingdon, Oxon OX14 4RN

Tel.:   +44 (0) 20 7017 6000
Fax.:   +44 (0) 20 7017 6699
E-mail: info.medicine@tandf.co.uk
Website: http://www.tandf.co.uk/medicine

A CIP record for this book is available from the British Library.

Library of Congress Cataloging-in-Publication Data

Data available on application

ISBN 1-84184-478-0
ISBN 978-1-84184-478-7

Distributed in North and South America by
Taylor & Francis
2000 NW Corporate Blvd
Boca Raton, FL 33431, USA

With Continental USA
Tel.: 800 272 7737; Fax.: 800 374 3401
Outside Continental USA
Tel.: 561 994 0555; Fax.: 561 361 6018
E-mail: orders@crcpress.com

Distributed in the rest of the world by
Thomson Publishing Services
Cheriton House
North Way
Andover, Hampshire SP10 5BE, UK
Tel.: +44 (0)1264 332424
E-mail: salesorder.tandf@thomsonpublishingservices.co.uk

Composition by Wearset Ltd, Boldon, Tyne and Wear

Printed and bound in Great Britain by TJ International Ltd, Padstow, Cornwall

Contents

Foreword	vii
Dedication	viii
Introduction	ix
List of abbreviations	xi
Abdominoplasty	1
Acute burns	3
Basal cell carcinoma	9
Botulinum toxin	12
Breast augmentation	15
Breast reconstruction	19
Breast reduction	23
Burn dressings	26
Burn surgery	30
Chemical burns	33
Cleft lip	36
Cleft palate	39
Complications	43
Craniosynostosis	49
Dupuytren's disease	52
Ear reconstruction	55
Electrical burns	58
Extensor tendon injuries	61
Facial anatomy	65
Facial lacerations	69
Facial reanimation	72
Flexor tendon injuries	75
Fractures of the mandible	82
Gynaecomastia	86
Hair removal	89
Hypoplastic facial conditions	92
Hypospadias	95
Informed consent	98
Keloids and hypertrophic scarring	100
Lasers: principles	103
Leg ulcers	107
Liposuction	110
Local anaesthetics	113
Lymphoedema	117
Melanoma	121
Microsurgery and tissue transfer	126
Neck dissection	129
Necrotizing fasciitis	134
Neurofibromatosis	136
Oral cancer	138

Paediatric burns 142
Parotid gland tumours 146
Premalignant lesions 150
Pressure sores 152
Prominent ears 155
Rhinoplasty 158
Skin grafts 161
Squamous cell carcinomas 164
Stevens–Johnson syndrome 166
Suturing 169
Tattoo removal 172
Tissue expansion 175
Ultraviolet light 177
Vacuum wound closure 179
Vascular anomalies 181
Zygomatic fractures 185

Index 188

Foreword

Within the past several decades, we have entered a period in the history of plastic and reconstructive surgery in which there has been a rapid development of subspecialties. The abundance of information generated from established or new ideas, concepts, knowledge, technology and techniques is difficult to assimilate, especially for medical students, nurses, general practitioners and plastic surgery trainees. It is, therefore, important for such groups to be provided with several key topics with broad current coverage written in a simple and readable manner.

Tor Chiu, Assistant Professor in Plastic and Reconstructive Surgery, Chinese University of Hong Kong, has authored this book 'Key Topics in Plastic and Reconstructive Surgery' with Professor Andrew Burd, based on the teaching at the university and its hospital. All chapters provide a succinct guide to a core topic of plastic and reconstructive surgery. The relevant content, the clear descriptions and lists of important points make this book unique and valuable. Doctors Tor Chiu and Andrew Burd are to be congratulated for their great contribution to education in the field of plastic and reconstructive surgery.

Fu-Chan Wei, M.D., F.A.C.S.
Professor, Plastic and Reconstructive Surgery
Dean, Medical College
Chang Gung University

獻給我的親愛父母

To my loving parents

Introduction

This book came about from the teaching of plastic and reconstructive surgery, making it fundamentally different from many books currently available that are essentially a set of revision notes that, comprehensive as they may be, are most useful to the person who wrote them. In addition, rather than have long lists and collections of isolated facts, we have tried to use clear descriptive prose to explain important points and concepts, using lists only where appropriate.

Further reading has been included, but this does not equate to the endorsement of the views or opinions expressed in the individual papers. We wish to encourage discussion. The systematic critical evaluation of an article is an important skill to acquire.

We hope that our approach allows the book to find a broader appeal. We have aimed for readability and succinctness in our explanations of key topics in this sub-specialty.

Tor Wo Chiu

Abbreviations

5FU	5-fluorouracil
ABI	ankle brachial index
AP	anteroposterior
ATLS	Advanced Trauma Life Support
BAPN	beta-aminopropionitrile
BCC	basal cell carcinoma
BCG	Bacille–Calmette–Guerin vaccination for tuberculosis
CFNG	cross-facial nerve grafting
CL	cleft lip
CL/P	cleft lip with or without associated cleft palate
CNS	central nervous system
CP	cleft palate
CSF	cerebrospinal fluid
CT	computed tomography
DD	Dupuytren's disease
DIEP	deep inferior epigastric perforator
DIPJ	distal interphalangeal joint
DNA	deoxyribose nucleic acid
DVT	deep vein thrombosis
ECG	electrocardiogram
EM	erythema multiforme
EMG	electromyogram
EMLA	eutectic mixture of local anaesthetics
ENT	ear, nose and throat
ER	extensor retinaculum
FDA	Food and Drug Administration
FDP	flexor digitorum profundus
FDS	flexor digitorum superficialis
FFP	fresh frozen plasma
FNAC	fine needle aspiration cytology
FTSG	full-thickness skin graft
HBO	hyperbaric oxygen
HIV	human immunodeficiency virus
HLA	human leukocyte antigens
HPV	human papilloma virus
ICP	intracranial pressure
ICU	intensive care unit
IGF	insulin-like growth factor
IgG	immunoglobin G
IJV	internal jugular vein
IMF	intermaxillary fixation
INR	international normalized ratio
KA	keratoacanthoma
LD	latissimus dorsi
MALT	mucosa-associated lymphoid tissue
MCPJ	metacarpophalangeal joint

MGH	Massachusetts General Hospital
MM	malignant melanoma
MRI	magnetic resonance imaging
MRND	modified radical neck dissection
MRSA	methicillin resistant *Staphylococcus aureus*
NA	needle aponeurectomy
ND	neck dissection
NF	necrotizing fasciitis
NF1	neurofibromatosis type 1
NICE	National Institute for Clinical Excellence
OPG	orthopantomogram
ORIF	open reduction and internal fixation
PCR	polymerase chain reaction
PCWP	pulmonary capillary wedge pressure
PDE	phosphodiesterase
PDGF	platelet-derived growth factor
PDS	polydioxanone suture
PE	pulmonary embolism
PIPJ	proximal interphalangeal joint
PSA	pleomorphic salivary adenoma
PUVA	psoralen ultraviolet A
QS	Q-switched
QSRL	Q-switched ruby laser
RFFF	radial forearm free flap
RND	radical neck dissection
RSTL	relaxed skin tension line
SCC	squamous cell carcinoma
SJS	Stevens–Johnson syndrome
SNB	sentinel node biopsy
SPE	streptococcal pyrogenic exotoxins
SPF	sun protection factor
SSD	silver sulphadiazine
SSG	split skin graft
TCS	Treacher–Collins syndrome
TEN	toxic epidermal necrolysis
TFL	tensor fascia lata
TGF	transforming growth factor
TNM	tumour node metastasis
TPA	tissue plasminogen activator
TPN	total parenteral nutrition
TRAM	transverse rectus abdominis myocutaneous
USG	ultrasonogram
VAMP	vesicle associated membrane protein
VF	ventricular fibrillation
VPI	velopharyngeal incompetence
XP	xeroderma pigmentosa
YAG	yttrium-aluminium-garnet
ZF	zygomaticofrontal

Abdominoplasty

Abdominoplasty, in general terms, is the surgical removal of excess skin and fat from the anterior abdominal wall. When patients present (typically after multiple pregnancies), it is important to assess their individual problem(s) systematically:

- excess fat
- excess skin
- divarication of the muscles of the abdominal wall
- abdominal striae and scars.

The ideal patient would be within the weight limits for their height with only a moderate abdominal fullness and would not be considering future pregnancies.
Abdominal fat is arranged in layers:

- a superficial layer that is uniformly compact with many dense fibrous septa
- a deep layer that is less organized with fewer septa and is primarily responsible for the abdominal contour.

Procedures

- **Abdominoplasty.** With a long suprapubic incision, a large flap of skin and fat is raised and undermined to the costal margin. The flap is then pulled downward and the excess tissue is excised. Repositioning of the umbilicus through the flap is required. There are some variations in placement and design of the scar, but the incision is generally placed low for cosmesis.
- **Mini-abdominoplasty.** This can be performed for excess tissue that lies below the umbilicus. As it involves only modest trimming with a smaller scar and obviates the need to reposition the umbilicus, it is a less extensive procedure overall but probably less effective too.

Supplementary procedures

- **Liposuction**, particularly suction-assisted liposuction (SAL), can be used to remove fat in patients without significant excess skin or as an adjunct to surgical procedures. It is used most often on the flanks; when combined with an abdominoplasty, it is particularly important to avoid damaging the blood vessels through excessive liposuction as this would jeopardize the skin flaps.
- **Plication of the recti** may be required if there is severe divarication. Plication around the umbilicus itself is avoided to prevent strangulation. Plication of the external oblique muscle has also been advocated. The procedure has a long lasting effect as demonstrated by postoperative CT scans (at six months) in some studies. Pregnancy after plication may cause potential problems.
- **A fleur-de-lis-shaped incision** (or inverted T) can deal with lower central abdominal fullness. It can be used to tighten the waist at the expense of an additional vertical scar.

Complications

Severe complications (e.g. pulmonary embolism and deep vein thrombosis) are very rare. Minor complications are more common (12%); these mainly involve:

- haematoma/seroma 6%
- infection/dehiscence/necrosis (including the umbilicus), 5–7%
- scar problems—hypertrophic scarring is common
- decreased sensation, 'dog ears'.

Contraindications

- smoking
- morbid obesity
- cardiovascular disease
- diabetes
- thromboembolic disease.

It was previously thought that supra-umbilical scarring would be a relative contraindication and such scarring was associated with an increase in complication rates (23% vs 7%, commonly fat necrosis) in one study. However, recent work suggests that with carefully selected patients, abdominoplasty may still be performed if the following are avoided: excessive tension during closure, over-dissecting the flap (especially laterally) and excessive concomitant liposuction. Pregnancy is not absolutely contraindicated, but there needs to be careful observation, particularly if plication of the recti has been performed.

Umbilicus

The aesthetics of a 'natural looking' umbilicus are subjective, changing with time and fashion, but the general consensus is that a vertically orientated umbilicus with a superior hood and slight surrounding fullness is most desirable. There are different types of incision to create the desired shape, e.g. reverse omega or 'smiley'. De-fatting of the midline to recreate the effect of a raphe is advocated by some.

The umbilical stalk needs to be positioned through the flap: the normal position of the umbilicus is level with the top of the iliac crest. Traditionally the umbilicus is tacked to the anterior rectus sheath. This has been reported to cause discomfort and consequently some have suggested tacking to the superficial fascia instead.

Further reading

El-Khatib HA, Bener A. Abdominal dermalipectomy in an abdomen with pre-existing scars: a different approach. *Plast Reconstr Surg* 2004; **114:**992–7.

Related topic of interest

- Liposuction.

Acute burns

Definition

A burn is damage caused by pathological excesses of energy within the tissues. This can occur through a number of mechanisms but for the purposes of this chapter, we will limit the discussion to thermal burns. Heat causes protein denaturation at 43°C and cell damage at 45°C. Burn injuries lead to the release of inflammatory mediators that increase capillary permeability—the fluid shift that then occurs may lead to hypovolaemic shock and death.

Jackson's burn model

This theoretical model of burn injury divides the tissue damage into zones depending on the distance from the contact area and is helpful in appreciating the dynamic and three-dimensional nature of a burn:

- **Zone of coagulation.** Tissue at the contact area is dead.
- **Zone of stasis.** Adjacent tissue is hypoperfused and oedematous and in a precarious condition; with adequate resuscitation to improve perfusion, it may recover, but continuing inflammation, superimposed infection or ischaemia can cause irreversible damage.
- **Zone of hyperaemia.** Tissue furthest away is minimally injured and will recover quickly (in 7–10 days).

Effective burns management aims to maximize the survival of tissue in the zone of stasis.

Types of thermal burn

- **scald**—caused by hot liquids or gases, such as a cup of tea
- **flame burn**—caused by burning of clothing or a flammable liquid on the skin
- **flash burn**—caused by explosions, e.g. an ignited gas leak
- **contact burn**—caused by physical contact with a hot object, e.g. an iron or radiator
- **radiation burn**—caused by close proximity to a heat source.

The depth of a burn is related to the energy transferred, which is related to the temperature of the agent and the contact time. This is modified by the thickness of the skin which is related to the patient's age as well as the anatomical site.

First aid

The aim of first aid is to reduce the ongoing damage by shortening the exposure to heat; this involves:

- **Removing the source** by extinguishing the flames, e.g. by rolling along the ground (**'stop, drop and roll'**), by using blankets, water or fire extinguishers as appropriate. Clothing that was burnt or soaked in the hot liquid retains heat and should be removed immediately.

- **Cooling the burnt skin** for 10 min or until the pain stops, but being watchful for hypothermia (**'cool the burn, warm the patient'**). Cooling a burn has been shown to be effective in increasing perfusion and reducing protein denaturation in the injured area if done within 30 min. After 3 h, this has no value other than reducing pain. Do not use ice.

Primary survey 'ABC'

Initial treatment should follow standard advanced trauma life support (ATLS) algorithms.

- **Airway**—cervical spine stability needs to be maintained. Open and maintain the airway; intubation may be required. Upper-airway oedema may cause obstruction; circumferential full-thickness burns of the neck may also cause extrinsic compression.
- **Breathing**—100% O_2 is given. Life-threatening injuries such as tension pneumothorax, massive haemothorax and massive flail chest can result from the initial incident, e.g. the force of the blast, or from injuries sustained while escaping the scene, such as jumping from a height. Circumferential full-thickness chest burns may limit ventilatory movements.
- **Circulation**—treat any life-threatening haemorrhage. Obtain adequate intravenous access.

Take an 'AMPLE' history:	The history is very important:
• **A**llergies • **M**edication • **P**ast medical history • **L**ast meal • **E**vent.	**Cause**—determines likely depth of the injury. **Place**—particularly if in an enclosed space, to ascertain risk of smoke inhalation. Enquire about any first aid given. There may be associated injuries from the initial event or from trying to escape.

Inhalational injury

Inhalational injury is a major cause of death in large burns. It may be classified according to the site of injury:

- **Supraglottic**—hot gases injure the upper airway directly, causing oedema. The obstruction may be delayed for up to 1–2 days and can resolve spontaneously after a few days.
- **Subglottic**—thermal injury to the distal airway is rare but chemical injury can be caused by noxious or irritant gases, such as acids or aldehydes.
- **Systemic**—inhaled gases may cause metabolic upset, e.g. carbon monoxide or cyanide compounds. Carboxyhaemoglobin levels can be measured (threshold is higher in smokers, 10% vs 5%), but depends on the time elapsed since the injury (half life 2–6 hours depending on which study you believe) and also on the oxygen delivered.

A high index of suspicion of possibility of an inhalational injury is required; intubating prophylatically is preferable to performing emergency intubation for overt respiratory distress. There are certain markers of potential inhalational injury; two or more indi-cate an increased risk:

- history of burn in an enclosed space
- singed nasal hairs
- burns or soot in oral cavity or pharynx
- hoarseness or other change in voice.

Endoscopic examination may provide direct evidence of upper-airway injury.

Secondary survey

The secondary survey involves a head-to-toe examination to look for other injuries:

- remove clothing
- examine for wounds
- assess area and depth of burn.

The neurological status is assessed by the patient's responses using the Glasgow coma scale or the simpler AVPU system (Alert, responsive to Voice, responsive to Pain or Unconscious). Remember to assess the pupil reflexes.

Temporary dressings for burns are simple; they should be clean (not necessarily sterile), moist and cool to reduce pain (but keep the patient warm). Clingfilm or saline-soaked gauze is perfectly adequate as a temporary dressing. No topical antiseptics/antibiotics are required at this stage.

Specific assessment of burns

Depth

Assessing the depth of a burn is important as it is the major determinant of healing and thus the likelihood of scarring. The healing potential lies in the appendigeal structures in the dermis. The commonest classification used is descriptive: the burn is either **full thickness** (involving whole epidermis and dermis) or not full thickness, i.e. **partial** (Table 1). Partial-thickness burns can be subdivided into superficial or deep, depending on the depth of dermal involvement. Assessment is relatively subjective (generally regarded as being accurate in only two-thirds of cases) and is dynamic—the burn has the potential to change, particularly in the first 2–3 days, and particularly if inotropes are used during resuscitation or if resuscitation is inadequate. Scalds are more likely to be heterogeneous in burn depth i.e. mixed depth.

- **Pinprick or test scratch** to test sensation as well as bleeding is sometimes used as a supplemental test for assessing burn depth.
- **Punch biopsy** is the most accurate test, but the significant processing time and expense required make it impractical. It would leave scars in non-full-thickness burns.
- **Laser Doppler imaging (LDI)** used to assess tissue blood flow is a simple, non-invasive way to determine burn depth, but it is expensive and relatively unwieldy for routine use.

Table 1 Features associated with different depths of burn.

Description	Colour and texture	Blisters	Capillary refill	Sensation/ pain	Healing
Very superficial (not really a 'burn') '1st degree'	Pink and dry	No	Rapid	Very painful, intact sensation	Involves epidermis only. Peels after a few days and heals without scarring
Superficial dermal	Pink/red, wet under blisters, may be oedematous	may be present (small)	Present	Extremely painful, sensate	Good potential for healing in 7–10 days
Deep dermal	Red/pale with fixed staining, thick oedema	may be present (bigger)	Impaired	+/−	Re-epithelializes from residual dermal elements but may take more than 2 weeks. Risk of problem scarring
Full thickness	White, pale or black, leathery	No	No	No	No healing possible. Scar/ contraction

Area

The severity of the injury is usually approximated to the burn surface area (BSA) as a percentage of the total body surface area, though this does not take into account the burn depth or any pulmonary injuries. In crude terms, the larger the burn, the more severe the injury, and the greater the degree of inflammatory response to fluid shift from the intravascular compartment to the tissues—hence the burn surface area is used to assess the risk of developing hypovolaemic shock.

- The body is divided into regions of 9% total body surface area (head and neck, upper limbs) or 18% (lower limbs, front of trunk and back of trunk) and 1% (perineum).
- **Wallace's rule of nines** is easy to remember, but is only an approximation (it tends to overestimate the size of the burn). It is unsuitable for children (different body proportions), except when modified.
- **Patient's palm** area (the palmar surface of both the anatomical palm and the closed fingers) is taken as 1% of the total body surface area. This is good for patchy burns, but is only an approximation (the area is nearer 0.8% of the body area). This method is not suited for burns larger than 10% of the total body surface area.

- Burns charts, e.g. the **Lund and Browder chart**, take account of different body proportions with age and provide a permanent visual record of the area and the depth of the burn.

Erythema (associated with first-degree burns) is not included in the assessment as it represents intra-epidermal damage with little irreversible damage or pathological insult, and heals without scarring.

Resuscitation

Inflammation increases the capillary protein permeability, leading to fluid shifts that decrease the circulating volume. Intravenous resuscitation is commenced when the body surface area burnt exceeds 15% in adults and 10% in children; these thresholds are rather arbitrary, but correspond to the dividing line between minor and moderately severe burns. Below the threshold, oral fluids would be expected to be adequate.

The Parklands formula

Resuscitation volume V (ml) $= 4 \times BSA$ (%) $\times$ body weight (kg)
The calculated volume is given over 24 h: half over 8 h and the remainder over 16 h. (BSA = percentage body surface area burnt)

Maintenance fluids are needed for children.

Most modern formulae are equally effective. They serve only as guides and require adjustment according to the patient's response. The single best measure in uncomplicated burns is the urine output (aim for more than 0.5 ml of urine per hour per kg). Typically, more fluids are needed with inhalational injuries, electrical burns or for those with concomitant crush injuries—osmotic diuresis may need to be encouraged using mannitol. No colloid is necessary in the first 24 h when the capillary permeability to macromolecules is highest.

Patient monitoring should include blood pressure (insensitive), pulse rate (non-specific) and temperature (the core–peripheral gradient can be used to gauge the peripheral perfusion). If required, the central venous pressure (CVP) and pulmonary capillary wedge pressure (PCWP) may be measured, but this necessitates invasive monitoring.

Other factors

Decompression
Fluid shifts cause tissue oedema, which, combined with loss of soft tissue elasticity after deep circumferential burns, may lead to raised compartment pressures. This is a surgical emergency.

- airway obstruction with neck burns
- breathing problems with thoracic burns
- compartment syndrome with limb burns.

Decompression is required: incision of the burn (escharotomy) may be adequate, but a deeper decompression in the form of fasciotomy is occasionally required. These procedures are best performed under controlled conditions in the operating room, with general anaesthesia and diathermy. There are guidelines for the preferred lines of incision, with particular care taken to avoid nerve damage.

Nutrition

Adequate feeding is important for healing and resistance to infection. When a burn is large, the daily calorific requirement can increase 1.5–1.75 times above normal. In more severe burns, a feeding tube should be inserted to decompress the gut and commence feeding, preferably within 8 h. Many formulae are available to calculate the increased calorific requirement, e.g. Harris-Benedict and Curreri. The use of vitamin supplements is advocated by some, but the role of such supplements in those who were previously healthy is unproven.

Total parenteral nutrition (TPN) is not indicated in acute burns and is in fact associated with a higher mortality rate; enteral feeding is preferred as it preserves gut integrity, reduces bacterial translocation and is safer with fewer complications.

Pain relief

Adequate pain relief is important. Keeping the patient comfortable will reduce catabolic requirements. Opiates are best given intravenously as absorption from intramuscular administration is unpredictable. Additional analgesia should be given before dressing changes.

Infection

Burn patients are at risk of infection, but prophylactic antibiotics are generally not given.

There is a decrease in both cellular and humoral immunity:

- decreased total lymphocyte numbers
- prolonged survival of allografts
- reduction of immunoglobulin levels
- serum from burn patients is immunosuppressive in vitro.

Dressings with physical cleansing of the wound and the use of tropical antimicrobials are the mainstay of reducing infection. Tetanus prophylaxis is given depending on the patient's immunization status.

Further reading

Herndon DN (ed.). *Total burn care.* London: WB Saunders, 1995.
The Australia and New Zealand Burns Association. *Emergency management of severe burns* (EMSB), course manual. Sydney: Australia and New Zealand Burns Association, 1996.

Related topics of interest

- Burns dressings
- Burns surgery
- Chemical burns
- Paediatric burns.

Basal cell carcinoma

Basal cell carcinoma (BCC) is the commonest human malignancy in Caucasians, it is less common in those with pigmented skin. The incidence varies from over 1500 in 100 000 in Queensland, Australia, to 200–300 per 100 000 in the United Kingdom, and 2–3 per 100 000 in Hong Kong Chinese. There is a male predominance, but the incidence in females is increasing.

The tumour arises in hair-bearing skin, particularly on the face where sun exposure is the highest; over three-quarters arise on the face, one-quarter on the nose. The lesion is generally slow-growing, but is locally destructive, hence the common name of 'rodent ulcer'.

Despite their name, BCCs probably do not arise from the basal cells of the epidermis but from the pluripotential cells in the epidermis; this is supported by the occasional observation of appendigeal differentiation in these tumours. The typical features are raised pearly edges and telangiectasia (small blood vessels) with or without a central ulcer. Histologically, there are undifferentiated cells in nodules with peripheral palisading ('picket fence pattern').

There are a number of morphological subtypes of BCC:

- Nodular—less than 5% of BCCs in Caucasians are pigmented (can look very similar to malignant melanoma), but pigmented carcinomas are more common in darker-skinned races. (Three-quarters of BCCs in Chinese patients are pigmented)
- Superficial—commoner on the trunk. Multiple lesions in a patient should raise the possibility of arsenic poisoning as a cause
- Morpheaform/sclerosing—often a scar-like lesion with ill-defined margins
- Infiltrative.

The latter two subtypes are more aggressive in behaviour. The overall rate of metastasis is extremely low but there have been several reports in the literature.

Sun exposure (ultraviolet B)—the strongest association is repeated sunburn in childhood with a lag time of 20–50 years; the field effect is demonstrated by the almost 50% risk of developing a further BCC in the subsequent 5 years. Psoralen ultraviolet A (PUVA) treatment for psoriasis is another risk factor.

Other risk factors include:

- immunosuppression
- exposure to carcinogens such as hydrocarbons/arsenic (occupational, medicinal or environmental—contaminated water supplies are often implicated)
- irradiation
- genetic conditions such as xeroderma pigmentosa or syndromes such as Gorlin's syndrome. It has a multitude of alternative names, including BCC syndrome which is inherited in an autosomal dominant manner. Patients have a predisposition to developing carcinomas from puberty onward,

particularly BCCs. Other associated feature include jaw cysts, bifid ribs, pits in the palms and soles, prominent brow with hypertelorism, partial agenesis of the corpus callosum with learning difficulties.

- pre-existing sebaceous naevus.

Treatment

Surgical excision is the standard treatment. Randomized trials of excision margins are lacking, but generally margins of 2 mm (for well-circumscribed lesions, particularly on the face) to 5 mm (for lesions with indistinct margins) are recommended. Four millimetre margins give a cure rate of 94–96% according to Zitelli.

Some areas such as the medical canthus, and external auditory alar base meatus are more prone to incomplete excision as the tumour seems to extend deeper at these locations; the usual explanation being that these areas are embryological fusion lines. Note that only one-third of incompletely excised BCCs will show histological evidence of residual tumour on further resection. Recurrent lesions tend to be more aggressive in behaviour.

Mohs' micrographic surgery (MMS)—in which successive layers are exised and the base of the specimen is mapped out and examined histologically perioperatively—may be most useful in complex lesions with indistinct borders and where tissue conservation is important. It has the best reported cure rate of 99%.

Other treatments

- Curettage with or without electrodesiccation. The lesion is scooped out piecemeal and the base is then usually cauterized (this adds little in the way of oncological clearance but causes most of the tissue damage leading to scarring). The recurrence rate is around 10%, however there is a lack of uniform protocols, and there is no margin information. The wound heals by secondary intention typically producing a white atrophic scar.
- Cryotherapy with liquid nitrogen (−50°C) has a comparable 10% recurrence rate, but no histological information is available.
- Radiotherapy is an effective alternative primary treatment for superficial BBCs. Better cosmesis can be achieved with fractionation regimes.
- Newer treatments
  —Aldara (5% imiquimod, 3M Pharmaceuticals) is an immune response modifier that results in a non-specific activation of the immune response; it is said to increase the production of cytokines, especially interferons. It is applied topically for six weeks and has an 85% response rate. It has recently gained FDA approval for the treatment of superficial tumours, in addition to actinic keratosis and genital warts.
  —Photodynamic therapy, with laser or non-laser light energy, is used to activate a photoactivated chemical that has been applied or injected. Metvix (methyl aminolevulinate 16%) is applied as a cream, the chemical is taken up by malignant cells and converted to porphyrins that are then activated by red light (570–670 nm). Due to the limited depth of penetration of tissue by light, only very superficial lesions are suitable for treatment. Treatment is usually repeated after a week. The overall response rate is 85% in selected lesions.

—Interferon and BCG vaccine injections have been described.

These alternatives can be considered for selected cases, particularly for superficial tumours, but are not recommended for treatment of aggressive subtypes (infiltrative and morpheaform) or recurrent cases.

Further reading

Snow SN, Sahl W, Lo JS et al. Metastatic basal cell carcinoma. Report of five cases. *Cancer* 1994; **73:**328–35.

Related topics of interest

- Melanoma
- Squamous cell carcinomas
- Ultraviolet light.

Botulinum toxin

Clostridium botulinum is a spore-forming, gram-positive, anaerobic rod. A number of different potent neurotoxins (from A–G) are produced by different strains. The name is derived from the Latin for sausage, *botulus*, due to its association with food poisoning from bad sausages. Botulinum toxin A is the most widely studied; it is the easiest to obtain from culture and was the first to be commercially prepared as Botox (Allergan). The toxin, consisting of two subunits (light and heavy chains are connected by a disulphide bridge), selectively inhibits acetylcholine release at the neuromuscular junctions in a dose-dependent manner.

Rhytides

Wrinkles (rhytides) are partly due to the contraction of underlying muscles and partly due to a loss of elasticity, thus paralyzing the muscles with the toxin will reduce wrinkles. The effect of toxin A on glabellar lines was noted incidentally when it was used therapeutically for strabismus and torticollis, and it subsequently gained FDA approval specifically for the treatment of glabellar lines. There is extensive use in cosmetic surgery for a wide variety of indications, generally in an 'off label' manner, as the indications for which the toxin is specifically licensed are fairly limited. Botulinum toxin is also used in conditions such as dystonias (blepharospasm and hemifacial spasm) or hyperhidrosis (excess sweating) in the axilla or face (Frey's syndrome).

The commonest areas treated with botulinum toxin are shown in Table 1.

Other areas include: lower and upper eyelid wrinkles, circumoral lines (orbicularis oris), nasal lines (nasalis), marionette folds or drooping labial commissure, chin folds or cobblestone chin (mentalis), platysmal folds or turkey neck, and decollete folds.

The toxin (about 5 U per site for Botox—more is needed in men due to greater muscle mass) is injected into muscle; some use EMG guidance. The action is delayed for 1–3 days because the toxin needs to be internalized and cleaved to take effect. The effects peak at 1–2 weeks and last for 8–12 weeks (if boosted, effects may last up to 9 months and may be due in part to muscle atrophy).

Table 1 Common areas treated with botulinum toxin.

Wrinkle	Underlying muscle
Glabella (vertical frown lines)	Corrugator supercilii, medial portion of orbicularis oculi, procerus, depressor supercilii
Forehead (horizontal frown lines)	Frontal belly of the occipitofrontalis
Periorbital/lateral canthus (crows' feet)	Lateral part of orbicularis oculi

Mechanism of action

At the molecular level, botulinum toxin A produces presynaptic inhibition at the neuromuscular junction:

- The toxin molecule binds to a specific receptor on cholinergic nerve endings.
- The toxin is internalized by receptor-mediated endocytosis and then cleaved into its constituent chains.
- The light chain is released into the cytoplasm and then cleaves SNAP-25 (synaptosomal-associated protein of 25 kDa) preventing the fusion of acetylcholine vesicles with the plasma membrane.
- Atonic paralysis of skeletal muscle (and also parasympathetic end organs) results and lasts until new synapses are formed by sprouting and new SNAP-25 is produced, reactivating the terminals.

A variety of commercial preparations that are currently available, are shown in Table 2.

The use of botulinum toxin is specifically contraindicated in areas of infection or in patients with prior allergic reactions to the toxin or its other constituents, e.g. albumin. In addition, caution is needed in:

- pregnant/lactating patients
- areas of inflammation

Table 2 Commercial preparations of botulinum toxin.

Trade name (manufacturer)	Storage	Notes
Botox (Allergan) toxin A	Lyophilized into crystals that need to be stored at −5°C. and reconstituted with 2.5–3 ml saline; usage within 4 h is recommended but effective in practice for up to 6 weeks	Four times more potent than Dysport. Reformulated after 1997 to a form that is said to have reduced problems with immunity
Dysport (Ipsen) toxin A	Powder reconstituted with saline can be stored at 2–8°C	Less potent unit per unit compared to Botox. Claims that it lasts longer but depends on dose given
Myobloc (Elan) US, also called Neurobloc in Europe toxin B	Solution. Can be stored in refrigerators for up to 20 months	Less potent than toxin A. Faster action: begins as early as 4 h, peaking at 2 weeks. Lasts half as long as toxin A. Affects synaptobrevin (vesicle associated membrane protein [VAMP]) in the synapse

- pre-existing neuromuscular disease, e.g. myasthenia gravis, Lambert–Eaton myasthenic syndrome
- concomitant use of neuromuscular drugs or anticoagulants. Aminoglycoside potentiates the effect of the toxin, whereas chloroquine reduces it.

In general, with careful use complications are rare; some experience headaches or a flu-like illness afterwards. The most common complication is temporary unwanted paralysis, e.g. ptosis is quoted at 3%; one should expect the toxin to diffuse within a 1.5 cm radius. Patients are advised to avoid massaging the area just after injection.

Bruising may occur, but is uncommon. As the toxin decreases the range of emotive expression, this may be an issue for actors (or politicians!). Immunity to the toxin due to antibodies is possible but rare (3–10%), and may lead to failure of the treatment. It is more common when multiple high doses are given, particularly as boosters. To avoid this, smaller doses given over a sufficiently long interval are used. Newer formulations are said to have fewer problems with immunity.

Further reading

Carruthers J, Fagon S, Matarasso SL, Botox Consensus Group. Consensus recommendations on the use of botulinum toxin type A in facial aesthetics. *Plast Reconstr Surg* 2004; **114**(6 Supp): 1S–22S.

Breast augmentation

Breast augmentation is a relatively common surgical procedure; it is estimated that 1% of US women have had augmentations. The vast majority of implants are used to enlarge breasts deemed too small by the patient; however, sometimes implants are used to reconstruct breasts after tumour resection (usually combined with latissimus dorsi flap) and less commonly in Poland's syndrome or in gender re-assignment surgery.

There are many options in terms of the type of implant, the type of access and the position in the chest wall that it occupies.

Types of implants

Material
- **Silicone.** Early silicone gels were liquid in nature, but currently favoured implants have a cohesive gel that is thicker and does not flow. It can be preformed in an anatomical shape and is supposed to have a smaller risk of leakage but does require a longer incision.
- **Saline.** In the US, only saline implants are available due to the FDA ruling in 1992, however these implants still have a silicone elastomer shell. They are associated with more rippling.
- **Soya oil.** Soya oil-filled implants are no longer available.

Envelope
- **Smooth** implants offer softer (better) consistency. However, the higher rate of capsule formation essentially restricts their positioning to the submuscular plane.
- **Textured** implants have an uneven surface that supposedly reduces formation of parallel lines of tension with multiple vectors that cancel each other out, and so reduce capsule formation. However, they may cause traction rippling, especially at the upper pole. The reported advantageous effect of texturing does not seem to be as marked in more recent studies, particularly for saline implants.
- Some earlier implants had a polyurethane shell that reduced capsule formation, but the material was shown to induce sarcomas in rats, and although there have been no reports in humans, their use was stopped. The recommendations are that existing implants need not be removed.

Shape
- Round or tear drop/anatomic—these are supposedly more breast-like with more fullness inferiorly, but studies have shown little difference in practice from conventional round implants. Shaped implants are usually textured to reduce rotation that would lead to an abnormal shape.

Placement

Submuscular
The rate of capsule formation seems to be reduced when implants are placed under muscle. The implant is placed under the chest wall muscles, which provide better

support of the implant and is associated with less visible and/or palpable rippling of the implant surface. The nerves are said to be less vulnerable to damage due to being less fixed in this region and there is less sensory disturbance. However, disadvantages include potentially increased bleeding due to the plane of dissection, muscle contraction potentially squeezing the implant into unattractive shapes and increased risk of the implant shifting in the pocket.

- Subpectoral, i.e. below pectoralis major only. The inferior pole is uncovered and only one-third to one-half is covered.
- Submuscular, below pectoralis major, serratus anterior laterally and the rectus abdominis fascia inferiorly. This is a less commonly used option.

Subglandular

Implants placed under the breast gland and above the muscle tend to fill the skin envelope better and, by occupying a 'proper' position, provide a more aesthetically pleasing result, particularly in moderate-sized breasts that are ptotic. However, the main disadvantages are a higher rate of capsule formation, and 'rippling' of the implant surface may be palpable or even visible. The implant may hinder mammography. It is relatively contraindicated in those who have undergone radiotherapy.

The clinical features of various types of access are given in Table 1.

Complications

Exact figures are difficult to come by as there are many different types of implant, and these may have undergone design changes at various stages.

Table 1 Clinical features of different types of access.

Type of access	Comments	Disadvantages
Inframammary	Good exposure, scar is mostly hidden in the field	A bigger scar
Periareolar incision	Scarring is minimal and usually well disguised	Risk of nipple paraesthesia is increased
Axillary	Less noticeable scar and does not cross breast tissue. Facilitated by endoscopic assistance and using inflatable implants	Decreased exposure. Scar may be visible when wearing sleeveless clothing. Risk of injury to intercostal brachii nerve and subclavian vein thrombosis
Transumbilical (TUBA— transumbilical breast augmentation)	Inflatable implant is tunnelled up to the breast. Scar is less noticeable	Longer operative time. Variable results

Early

Infection and haematoma/seroma occur in around 2–3% of cases. Bacteria have been occasionally found in implants, and this is usually attributed to contamination during the procedure.

Late

- Capsule formation (with modern implants is 10% over 3 years).
- Rupture (4–6% and usually due to trauma) is best detected with MRI (step-ladder sign) or ultrasound (requires experienced ultrasonographer).
- Microscopic gel bleed may occur, predisposing the patient to granulomas—newer implants are 'low bleed'. Scar tissue forms quickly around implants so silicone is usually not detectable more than 2 mm beyond the implant.
- Skin numbness is usually temporary.
- The implant position may be asymmetric or may become displaced.
- An implant may be palpable/visible especially in very thin patients; 'rippling' is a common cause of dissatisfaction.

Baker classification of capsular contracture

1. Normal implant
2. Palpable capsule
3. Visible distortion of implant
4. Painful implant.

The exact cause(s) of capsule formation are unclear, but possibly involve a foreign body reaction and/or low-level bacterial infection, especially of *Staphylococcus epidermidis*—for this reason, prophylactic antibiotics and local irrigation of the dissected pocket with betadine is advocated by some. Antibiotics have not been shown to consistently reduce capsule formation, but betadine does have a beneficial effect (12% vs 28% using saline irrigation) that is independent of the effect of texturing. Massage is encouraged by some, and while there are positive psychological benefits, the effect on capsule formation is largely unproven.

The most predictable way of **reducing capsule formation** is to place saline implants in a submuscular/subpectoral location. The effect of texturing is not as predictable. Capsules are generally treated with open capsulectomy/capsulotomy and implant exchange. Closed capsulotomy is not recommended as the forces involved exceed the breaking strength of the implant.

The safety of silicone breast implants

Silicone is a silicon–carbon-based polymer and had already been in use for many years in various medical devices, tubes and syringes when it was first used in breast implants in 1963 in the USA. In 1992, in response to reports that they cause cancer and autoimmune disease, the FDA ordered a moratorium on silicone implants for cosmetic use (their use in reconstruction was still allowed if part of an approved study).

However, the general consensus among professionals is that there is no correlation between silicone levels and connective tissue disease or cancer, and this is supported by many large-scale epidemiological studies. Ironically, patients with silicone implants have a reduced rate of breast cancer; this may be related to the smaller breast mass or a possible direct protective effect. Studies in rats suggest that this may be related to tissue expander effects on blood flow, and blood from implant patients kills cancer cells in situ.

Other issues

Mammography
Radio-opaque silicone and capsule formation/microcalcification may hinder the investigation, particularly if the implant is placed above the muscle. However, the general consensus is that as long as the radiologist is experienced with implants, mammography can still be satisfactory. The Eklund technique has a larger number of views and increases the amount of breast tissue revealed from 56% to 64% for subglandular placement of implants and from 75% to 85% for submuscular placement. Some recommend preoperative mammograms if the patient is over 35 years of age, and/or has a positive family history.

Breast feeding
A study found similar levels of silicone in breast milk in patients with (n = 6) or without implants, demonstrating the ubiquitous presence of silicone in the modern environment. In fact, cow's milk and infant formula contain more silicon than breast milk from women with implants.

Further reading

Nyren O, Yin L, Josefssen S et al. Risk of connective tissue disease and related disorders among women with breast implants: a nationwide retrospective cohort study in Sweden. *Brit Med J* 1998; **316:**417–22.

Breast reconstruction

The breast may be absent or malformed due to a congenital deficiency, or it may be disfigured as a consequence of disease or injury such as post-burn scarring. However the majority of reconstructions follow breast cancer surgery. The goal is to construct a breast that matches the normal contralateral breast in size, projection/contour and texture. In practice, natural ptosis and a good inframammary fold are difficult to achieve.

Post-cancer reconstruction

Most breast tumours are ductal (80%) or lobular (15%). Surgery is also offered for in situ disease detected on mammogram as a result of calcification (DCIS) or coincidentally on biopsy (LCIS). Breast cancer genes BRCA1 and 2 are found in around 5% of cases, along with mutations in tumour suppressor genes; the presence of BRCA1 and 2 is a likely finding if there are more than four cases under 60 years of age in a single family. Patients with the genes have an 85% lifetime risk of developing breast cancer.

Immediate or delayed reconstruction

Immediate reconstruction is often regarded as the gold standard as it diminishes the emotional upset after the diagnosis of cancer and mastectomy. In addition there are definite advantages: the skin flaps are more pliable and the inframammary fold is easier to maintain. The overall aesthetic result tends to be superior, with better ptosis and superior fullness compared with delayed reconstruction.

The concerns about immediate reconstruction are mainly oncological. Many surgeons feel that delay may be prudent if radiotherapy is necessary, although numerous studies have shown that immediate breast reconstruction does not interfere with adjuvant therapy, including radiotherapy, chemotherapy or hormonal therapy. Studies have also found that there is no delay in diagnosis of recurrent tumours. Thus immediate reconstruction has been shown to be oncologically safe, indeed some say safer, because further surgical trauma may cause immunosuppression and stimulate previously dormant tumour cells.

Breast reconstruction is in principle a 'cosmetic' procedure and therefore the patient's aesthetic demands will need to be balanced carefully with the surgical risks. A significant number will not want reconstruction, particularly if mastectomy has already been performed, as they do not wish to have the trauma of another major operation. However, it is the duty of the surgeon to advise of its availability.

No reconstruction

For many, a simple external prosthesis or padded bra is all that is required. For selected small tumours, lumpectomy may be performed through skin incisions used in breast reduction techniques; the opposite breast may need surgery to improve symmetry.

Implants alone

More commonly, implants are placed under a latissimus dorsi flap, which provides good quality vascularized soft tissue coverage. A tissue expander is placed under the muscle and inflated weekly until it is 'over-expanded' (approximately 30%) compared to the opposite side. At this point, the expander is exchanged for a slightly smaller prosthesis to create a degree of ptosis; in specially designed composite expanders (saline core within a silicone prosthesis), the expander also acts as the implant. After removing some saline to recreate ptosis, the filling port is removed if necessary.

Becker expander implant	McGhan expander implant
• 25% silicone (by final volume) • distant filling port can be pulled out.	• 50% silicone • integral filling port over implant located by magnet • has a fuller shape inferiorly, and thus needs to be textured to prevent rotation of the implant.

The insertion of an implant/expander is a relatively simple procedure with few serious complications, but numerous visits are involved. Being foreign bodies, implants or expanders can suffer from problems such as infection, extrusion and capsule formation but these complications may be reduced with submuscular positioning of the implant.

The use of implants is relatively contraindicated after irradiation of the chest wall because the skin and the muscle may not be capable of stretching sufficiently. Radiotherapy cannot be given while the expander is still being filled.

Pedicled flaps
• **Latissimus dorsi** (LD) is a very reliable flap. Its main disadvantage is that it usually requires an implant to recreate anything other than small breasts. The donor scar on the back is large and seromas are not uncommon. The skin of the LD flap is thicker and darker than the front of the chest, thus creating a patch effect. The flap may not be available if the thoracodorsal vessels were damaged during axillary dissection, although a flap can still be raised on the serratus anterior branch under some circumstances.
  —To reduce the need for an implant, an extended LD flap can be raised by taking more adjacent soft tissue, e.g. in a fleur-de-lis pattern, but the scar is longer and the distal tissue is less reliable.
• **TRAM** (transverse rectus abdominis myocutaneous) is usually pedicled on the contralateral superior epigastric artery. It is relatively contraindicated in the obese and in smokers. It can be 'supercharged' by anastomosing the deep inferior epigastric artery to the thoracodorsal artery or 'super-drained' to the veins to improve drainage.

Free flaps
Free flaps tend to produce the best breast shape in terms of projection and ptosis. However, there is the potential for complete flap loss (1–2%) and it requires microsurgical experience and equipment. The longer operating times and greater anaesthetic risk means that it may not be suited to those with medical problems.

- **TRAM**—the free flap is based on the stouter (deep) inferior epigastric artery, and consequently, the incidence of fat necrosis is much reduced compared to the pedicled flap. It can be anastomosed to the contralateral internal thoracic/mammary vessels (usually providing more transverse fullness) or the ipsilateral thoracodorsal artery (more vertical fullness). It cannot be used in those who have had previous abdominoplasty or liposuction. But the presence of a gynaecological Pfannenstiel scar (usually low and muscle splitting) does not preclude the use of the flap.
- **DIEP** (deep inferior epigastric perforator) Perforator flaps have the advantage of leaving the muscle mass and fascia behind, with less donor site morbidity, specifically in terms of the strength of trunk flexion on the hip and the incidence of hernias, although the difference may become less pronounced with time and specific training. Dissecting the vessel out of the muscle necessitates a longer operating time. The vessel is longer but thinner and the incidence of fat necrosis is slightly higher than for the TRAM flap; it may be more suited to cases where the flap needed is two-thirds or less of the TRAM flap area. A compromise is a muscle sparing TRAM.

Less common free flaps are used when TRAM/DIEP flaps are not available:

- **Superior gluteal artery** flaps provide reasonable shape but have a relatively short central pedicle and have potential donor problems with scarring and contouring. It may be raised as a perforator flap.
- **Inferior gluteal artery flaps** have longer pedicles and leave a less-obvious scar (though you have to sit on it). As the sciatic nerve is exposed during the dissection, it is theoretically at risk particularly from postoperative scarring and there is a variable functional loss associated with the division of the inferior gluteal nerve.
- **Lateral thigh flaps** good projection is possible due to the thick fat over the greater trochanter.
- **Deep circumflex iliac artery** ('Rubens') flaps use the soft tissue around the iliac crest. Closure of the abdominal wall must be meticulous.

Advantages of free flaps compared with pedicled flaps, e.g. TRAM:

- The inferior pedicle deep inferior epigastric is shorter and sturdier than the superior epigastric, therefore the free flap is more reliable and there is less fat necrosis. It can thus be used where a pedicled flap is relatively contraindicated, e.g. in the overweight, in smokers as well as in cases where the superior pedicle is unavailable due to previous surgery.
- Less muscle is taken, reducing the degree of abdominal wall dysfunction.
- A better-shaped breast mound is achieved without the medial fullness that results from the tunnelled pedicle, and shaping and insetting are not limited by tethering at the pedicle.

Further reading

Hussien M, Salah B, Malyon A, Wieler–Mithoff EM. The effect of radiotherapy on the use of immediate breast reconstruction. *Eur J Surg Oncol* 2004; **30:**490–4.

Related topic of interest

• Breast augmentation.

Breast reduction

The aim of breast reduction surgery (or reduction mammaplasty) surgery is to reduce breast size while maintaining the aesthetics (symmetry with minimal scarring) and function (nipple sensation, ability to breast feed). The commonest indication is back pain due to the muscular imbalance caused by excessive weight. Oversized breasts can cause significant psychological upset and embarrassment. Other problems include intertrigo, grooving of the shoulder from bra straps, having difficulty with sports or being unable to find suitable clothes to wear. Despite the significant scar and potential complications, patient satisfaction is generally high (95% of patients regard their surgery as successful). Patients consistently rate the results higher than surgeons.

Operative techniques

There are many techniques, each with their own pros and cons, and no single technique can be applied to all patients. The general surgical considerations are:

- type of pedicle to improve nipple survival as well as maximizing sensation
- type of skin incision/excision to deal with skin excess and improve the scar.

Dilute adrenaline (epinephrine) infiltration is routinely used to reduce blood loss and less than 1% of patients require transfusion. The use of vasoconstrictors is not associated with an increase in postoperative bleeding or any vascular compromise of the flaps.

Pedicles

The earliest reduction operation is credited to Thorek (1922), who amputated large breasts and then used a free graft for the nipple. The major problem was unpredictable nipple survival, and subsequent techniques, based on improved understanding of the skin supply, kept the nipple attached to the chest wall on a pedicle (glandular or dermoglandular) to improve nipple survival. Excess breast tissue is debulked *around* the pedicle.

There have been continual refinements in technique:

- One of the earliest techniques used **horizontal pedicles** (Strombeck) to improve nipple survival but had problems with reduced nipple sensation and tethering.
- Use of a **vertical pedicle** improved nipple perfusion without problems with tethering. The McKissock technique uses a superior dermal bridge to maintain the subdermal plexus in addition to an inferior dermoglandular pedicle to increase blood supply to the nipple and is regarded as a 'belts and braces' approach with good safety. However, the resultant breasts tend to have fullness superiorly with the nipples inclining downward.
- Subsequently, it was realized that the superior pedicle could be dispensed with safely, leading to **inferior pedicle** techniques (Robbins), which are the most widely used worldwide. It is a good versatile technique.
- Central mound techniques (Balch) dispense with the dermal pedicle and rely entirely on the parenchymal mound.

Nipple sensation is well-maintained in both superior and inferior pedicle techniques by preserving the anterior branch of the fourth lateral intercostal nerve in a generous wide mound because the nerve stays close to the muscle layer until mid-breast level.

Skin excision pattern
The most common pattern of skin excision is the Wise pattern, which removes a keyhole-shaped area of skin and results in an anchor-shaped scar.

With consistent nipple survival possible with pedicles, further modifications were aimed predominantly at improving the aesthetics.

- Lejour/Lassus vertical mammaplasty uses a superior pedicle and is popular due to the elimination of the inferior transverse scar and the provision of a longer-lasting attractive shape with good projection. Unfortunately, there is a steep learning curve and the puckering and shape may take weeks to months to settle. It is best avoided in those with excessive amounts of ptosis or redundant skin. There is a higher risk of nipple numbness in comparison to the inferior pedicle technique.
- Regnault B technique has an oblique scar that avoids a large medial component.
- Round block periareolar incision (Benelli) is similar to a mastopexy incision.

Postoperative care

- The use of drains is fairly common, although the practice is not wholly evidence-based.
- It is important to monitor nipple circulation and be alert to the possible formation of a haematoma (pain, swelling with hardening).
- Support. A surgical bra is worn for 2 weeks and then a sports bra for another 4–6 weeks; underwired bras are to be avoided. The bra band size will be unchanged.
- Pain with the first menstruation is not uncommon.
- Lactation is still possible in 70% of patients after using the inferior pedicle technique.

Complications

- Haematoma/wound infection/dehiscence.
- Skin necrosis/fat necrosis (the latter is probably more common than recognized).
- Nipple loss or numbness—reduced sensation occurs in around 5% of patients and is more frequent with more radical reductions. The biggest aesthetic mistake to make is to position the nipple too high.
- Shape—asymmetry 'bottoming out' of the vertical scar or 'dog ears' may require subsequent revision.
- Scar hypertrophy is not uncommon but can be reduced with treatment such as silicone therapy.

Alternatives to surgery

The use of liposuction alone for reduction is controversial; only 20% of the breast volume can be extracted by liposuction. In general, it is suitable only for a small proportion of patients; it may be useful in those with moderate-sized **fatty** breasts with **good skin tone** (as it can increase ptosis), or to make minor adjustments to improve symmetry after surgery. It does not remove parenchymal tissue and thus the risk of unknowingly removing malignant tissue is small.

Oncology

A very small number of patients who have breast reductions will turn out to have breast cancer: a quarter of these are found during preoperative assessment, another quarter as a result of perioperative 'suspicion' and half are found incidentally on routine pathological examination.

- Some recommend that those at moderately high risk of developing breast cancer (family history, age >35 years old—exact age is controversial) have a mammogram before surgery and a postoperative mammogram after 3–6 months as a baseline.
- Excised breast tissue is sent for histological examination with the sides marked carefully. There is a quoted 0.4% incidence of occult carcinoma in breast reduction specimens.

Postoperative changes result in calcification of breast tissue, but the mammographic appearance can usually be distinguished from malignant microcalcification.

Further reading

Jansen DA, Murphy M, Kind GM, Sands K. Breast cancer in reduction mammaplasty: case reports and a survey of plastic surgeons. *Plast Reconstr Surg* 1998; **102:**361–4.

Related topic of interest

- Liposuction.

Burn dressings

Properties of ideal burns dressing

Much has been written about the desirable properties for the 'perfect dressing', which does not exist. A good dressing should offer:

- Protection from further harm
  —desiccation
  —infection
  —mechanical trauma.
- Promotion of healing
  —promoting natural autolysis of the eschar (proteolysis and phagocytosis), which must occur prior to healing
  —providing an optimally moist environment; avoiding desiccation but must also deal with the wound exudate to avoid maceration.
- Pain relief.

First aid and dressings

Cooling a burn for 10–20 min is beneficial if performed within 30 min of the injury. It has been demonstrated to:

- reduce lactate production and acidosis
- reduce histamine release and oedema
- reduce thromboxane release and vascular occlusion.

For small burns, cooling can be continued after the 30 min for pain control, but with larger burns, continued cooling risks hypothermia. Remember to 'cool the burn, warm the patient'.

First aid dressings need only be clean (and not necessarily sterile) and wet (to reduce pain rather than cool the burn). Antiseptics or antimicrobials should be avoided at this stage.

Burns patients are prone to infection due to:

- open wound due to skin loss
- burn eschar with necrotic tissue
- use of invasive devices and procedures in their care
- immunosuppression (both cellular and humoral).

The commonest organisms infecting burns are *Pseudomonas aeruginosa* and *Staphylococcus aureus*. MRSA can be a difficult problem and toxic shock syndrome (TSS) is severe but thankfully rare. There is little role for systemic prophylaxis; antibiotics are generally given as indicated by culture results and patient condition.

Definitive dressings

Regimes are very variable and dictated largely by local practice. There are many alternatives to choose from and formal comparative studies are lacking. There are two basic aims of burns dressing:

- Reduce the risk of infection
- Optimize healing.

These are achieved by adjusting the dressing protocol in terms of:

- Extent of mechanical cleansing or debridement at dressing changes and the frequency of dressing changes. The aim of reducing infection by regular thorough scrubbing is balanced against maximizing healing by minimal disturbance to the delicate re-epithelializing wound. Local practice determines where the balance lies.
  —Analgesia, including opiates, should be given before dressing changes.
  —Warm tap water and soap can be used in simple burns; sterility is not essential. Saline for irrigation or chlorhexidine can be used for larger, deeper burns.
- Dressing material used.

Types of dressings

There is a wide choice of dressings available for burns:

- basic dressings—including gauze and tulle
- occlusive dressings
- antimicrobials—often based on silver
- skin substitutes.

Basic dressings

The earliest dressings were made of cloth. Cotton wool in its native state is non-absorbent due to surface oils, but bleaching increases its absorbency. Gamgee combines them with gauze covering cotton wool. A major problem with such dressings is adhesion to the wound bed; this is reduced by impregnating the gauze with paraffin oil to produce *tulle gras* (tulle is named after the French town famous for the fine net-like material). There is a variety of preparations with impregnated antiseptics/antibacterials that are in common use:

- Bactigras (0.5% chlorhexidine)
- Sofra Tulle (framycetin)
- Fucidin Intertulle (fusidic acid)
- Xeroform (3% bismuth tribromophenate).

Occlusive dressings

The aim is to promote healing by providing a moist environment. They are popular with patients as they can reduce pain and may not need to be changed everyday. This is a rather heterogeneous group of materials with their own advantages and disadvantages:

- hydrocolloids
- alginates (derived from seaweed) forms a gel when moistened and has haemostatic action, making it useful for dressing skin graft donor sites
- gels
- foams.

Antimicrobials

- Non-silver e.g. bactroban (mupirocin), neomycin and bacitracin. Sulfamylon (mafenide acetate) is a cream with a broad spectrum action with excellent penetration, including cartilage, making it useful for ear and nose burns. It can be painful, and carbonic anhydrase inhibition may cause alkaline diuresis and metabolic acidosis.
- Silver—many burns dressings are based on silver. Silver has a proven antimicrobial action but it is also potentially cytotoxic.

Silver nitrate
Silver nitrate (0.5%) has a broad antimicrobial action with minimal absorption and toxicity; however, it needs to be made up with distilled water and so can cause electrolyte loss due to hypotonicity. It is labour intensive to use because of the need for regular re-application/wetting, and in addition, it stains materials black.

Silver sulphadiazine (Flamazine)
Silver sulphadiazine (SSD) has a good action against gram negatives and gram positives including *Pseudomonas aeruginosa* with minimal pain, but systemic adsorption may lead to toxicity and to leucopaenia in particular (5–15%). Such leukopaenia is rarely profound and usually resolves in a few days without needing to stop the cream. It forms a pseudoeschar that may hinder depth assessment. However, SSD stimulates hydrolysis of burns by promoting inflammation and possibly more scarring; the increase in vascularity makes surgery more bloody. Its use should be avoided on the face. It has been the standard burns cream for many years and is still in wide use, although variants are becoming more popular as alternatives:

- flammacerium: SSD with cerium nitrate; this forms a firm eschar with less inflammation
- silvazine: SSD with 0.2% chlorhexidine to improve antimicrobial action.

Other silver dressings
- Acticoat and Silverlon are both silver-impregnated dressings that deliver silver ions to the wound.
- Aquacel silver is a hydrofibre dressing that aims to absorb bacteria along with wound exudate into the dressing where the silver ions kill bacteria. In this way, it aims to reduce silver toxicity.

Biological dressings
Cadaveric skin is regarded as the gold standard biological dressing but its use is hampered by lack of donors in certain cultures. It is available as:

- non-viable dressing when processed by gamma irradiation, glycerolization or lyophilization

- viable when stored in a fridge or in liquid nitrogen. With immunosuppression, it has the potential to be a true 'allograft', a skin transplant.

Dressings from animal skins are a reasonable substitute with greater availability; frog skin and porcine skin are the commonest.

Dressings from plants material may also be used, e.g. banana leaf and potato skin.

Biological dressings adhere to the wound without the need for staples, and except where they are being used as transplants, they will come off when re-epithelialization is complete. They relieve pain, have an antibacterial action and can be used in a variety of ways as a temporary dressing:

- to cover partial-thickness wounds to promote natural healing
- to cover debrided wounds while waiting for autograft
- to cover widely meshed autografts to keep interstices moist (sandwich grafting or Alexander technique). Usually cadaveric skin is used for this purpose.

Typical dressing regimes

Superficial partial-thickness burns will heal quickly, with little to choose between dressing types:

- Tulle gras (Jelonet) is the simplest.
- Moist wound healing provided by occlusive dressings and skin substitutes will provide faster healing.
- Antimicrobials are not necessary.

The burn wound is exudative in the first 48 h. Thus tulle gras or other absorbent dressing may be used first, followed by either occlusive dressings or skin substitutes.

Mixed/intermediate-depth wounds with significant eschar—dressing regimes must balance the risk of infection against the risk of desiccation.

- Occlusive dressing with non-silver antimicrobial
- Silver-based cream or dressing.

Full-thickness burns require excision, but can be dressed by antibiotic dressing while waiting for surgery.

- Silver-based dressings
- Other antimicrobials.

Further reading

Chiu T, Pang P, Ying SY, Burd A. Porcine skin: friend or foe? *Burns* 2004; **30:**739–41.

Related topics of interest

- Acute burns
- Burns surgery.

Burn surgery

The surgical management of the burn patient is determined to a large extent by the depth of the burn wound:

- When a burn is full thickness, it has to be excised with wound closure, unless it is very small in area.
- When a burn involves just the epidermis and superficial dermis, healing will take place in approximately 1 week.

Challenges arise when the burn depth falls into an intermediate category: a deeper dermal burn can heal, but the longer it takes to heal, the greater the chance that hypertrophic scarring will develop. Where healing is likely to take more than 2–3 weeks with significant risk of problem scarring (the risk is higher in pigmented races), surgery is needed to expedite healing and reduce scarring.

Early surgery

Early surgery to remove burn eschar has proven to be of benefit in the:

- removal of the source of inflammatory mediators
- removal of a potential site of infection.

Benefits in terms of reduced sepsis, mortality, hospital stay and costs have been demonstrated by many studies.

The exact definition of 'early' is not set in stone and varies between units. A reasonable working interpretation would be within 3–5 days, but basically, one should aim to operate:

- as soon as the patient is stable enough, and certainly
- before the wound is colonized
- before the hyperaemic stage (2–3 weeks).

Delayed surgery is indicated in cases of intermediate or mixed burn or in children with scalds (generally more heterogeneous or of 'mixed depth'), where the benefit of the doubt may be given for approximately 2 weeks.

Surgery

Heat loss particularly during surgery is a problem and the patient's temperature needs to be careful monitored. Burnt skin loses it thermoregulatory function, and operative exposure increases evaporative losses. The ambient temperature of the operating room is increased; other measures such as warming blankets may be used.

Blood loss is always a concern and is influenced by the method of excision:

- **Tangential excision** of eschar—The aim is to remove only the dead skin only by gradual shaving until viable tissue is indicated by bleeding, which may be significant.
  —Bleeding can be stopped by adrenaline (epinephrine)-soaked gauze and cautery. Limbs may be bandaged and elevated.

—Bleeding may also be reduced by infiltrating dilute adrenaline solution before surgery, but this may make judging the depth more difficult.

—Limb burns may be shaved under tourniquet control.

- **Fascial excision**—full-thickness or infected wounds can be excised along with subcutaneous tissue down to the fascia. Blood loss is much reduced and graft take is good but cosmesis is poor; lymphatic flow is reduced, leading to lymphoedema.

There are sound physiological reasons for total burn excision where possible. However, excision may be staged depending on local logistical support and the burn depth and size. Herndon advocates excising a maximum of 20% surface area on days 1, 3 and 5, while others suggest that 30% is the maximum that should be excised at one operation.

If staged, the general order is:

- hands and upper limbs
- lower limbs
- chest and back
- the face is usually left until last, except for the eyelids, which are a priority.

Hands require aggressive surgery to preserve function as much as possible.

- VAC (vacuum-assisted closure) dressings may be used to encourage the formation of granulation tissue.
- The palms rarely need grafting as the skin is thicker and it is protected by reflex closure.
- During and after treatment, it is vital to splint the hand in the position of function with metacarpophalangeal joints flexed, interphalangeal joints extended, thumb abducted and wrist extended.

Wound closure

Due to the large areas involved, full-thickness skin grafts typically are not used except under special circumstances, e.g. on the face in chemical burns.

Split-thickness skin grafts (SSG) are used either as a sheet (better cosmesis but at higher risk of developing collections) or meshed with a special machine that places holes at regular intervals allowing it to expand to cover a wider area. The mesh can be made in various ratios from 1:1.5 to 1:6 or more in rare circumstances, depending on the clinical requirements.

Meshing:
- increases the area that can be covered, and thus reduces the donor area required
- allows drainage of exudates/haematoma that may otherwise collect and reduce graft take.
- improves conformity of the graft to the contours of the wound.

However, meshing leaves a pattern even after healing, and with a wider mesh (e.g. 1:6), the interstices between the skin bridges are prone to dessicate before re-epithelialization from the sides can occur. Such widely meshed skin grafts would benefit from being covered with sheet allograft (sandwich technique) or cultured keratinocytes to protect the interstices from desiccation.

When insufficient unburnt skin is available for use:

- Temporary dressings may be used while waiting for the donor to heal for re-cropping. Re-cropping is limited by the dermal thickness as the dermis does not regenerate.
  —Cadaveric skin is often regarded as the gold standard temporary dressing, but suffers from limited supplies. There is a theoretical risk of viral transmission. Rejection/ejection can be delayed as a result of immunosuppression in major burns patients.
  —Animal skin (often called 'xenografts') works similarly to cadaveric skin. Pig and frog skin are the most commonly used.
- Skin substitutes may be used where skin is in short supply.
  —Integra (silicone covering over bovine collagen–glycosaminoglycans matrix).
  —Biobrane (silicone and nylon mesh with collagen).
- Another alternative is to culture the patient's own keratinocytes from a skin biopsy of approximately 2×2 cm, to form:
  —Sheets, which take up to 2–3 weeks. The new skin is fragile; the immature epidermal–dermal junction makes it prone to bulla formation.
  —Suspensions, which can be made quicker, can be used for widely meshed split skin grafts or to heal donor sites.

Further reading

Jackson DM, Stone PA. Tangential excision and grafting of burn. The method, and a report of 50 consecutive cases. *Br J Plast Surg* 1992; **25:**416–26.

Related topics of interest

- Burns dressings
- Skin grafts
- Vacuum wound closure.

Chemical burns

Chemical burns account for less than 5% of the admissions to most burns units. They are usually accidents (either at work or at home) or deliberate personal assaults. The severity of a burn depends on:

- nature of the agent
- concentration of the agent
- contact time.

In industry, even with high concentrations of chemicals, injuries tend to be minor, probably as a result of the greater awareness of the problem and the availability of facilities for rapid decontamination; whereas in the home or after assaults, contact can be prolonged and can cause potentially devastating damage.

Most chemical burns can be categorized as follows:

- acid
- alkali
- organic—e.g. hydrocarbons
- extravasation injuries.

First aid

Always take care.

- Remove the chemical from the patient. Immediately irrigate with cool water to dilute the chemical—there is never too much irrigation as long as the patient is kept warm. Running water is preferred to 'soaks' as it dissipates both the chemical and the heat of dilution more effectively. Be wary of causing damage to neighbouring regions with 'run-off'. pH paper can be used to guide the adequacy of treatment.
- 'Neutralization' with another chemical is generally not recommended as it would cause an exothermic reaction and the neutralizing agent itself may cause burns. There are certain situations in which water should be avoided:
  —Alkali metals (sodium, potassium and lithium) undergo exothermic reactions with water. The material should be covered with oil before gently wiping away.
  —The penetration of phenol increases with dilution. Polyethylene glycol wipes are better.
  —White phosphorous oxidizes in air and combines with water to produce phosphoric acid.
- Remove contaminated clothing.
- Remove jewellery.
- Trim fingernails.

Further management

- Continue irrigation as tolerated, using pain and wound pH as guides.
- Eye assessments—the eyes should be specifically checked. Thorough irrigation is required if the eyes are involved.

- Monitor for local and systemic effects, e.g. renal and liver failure; include arterial blood gas analysis to check for metabolic acid–base disturbance.

Acids

Acid burns can be very painful; they generally cause coagulative necrosis and protein denaturation.

- Hydrochloric/sulphuric acid are found in toilet cleaners.
- Formic acid is found in descalers and leaves a burn with a typical green colour with blisters.
- Hydrofluoric acid is found in cleaning agents and is used in glass manufacturing (etching). It is actually a weak acid; the danger comes from the fluoride ion causing hypocalcaemia and arrhythmias. In this way, a small burn can still be fatal. There is intense pain with progressive destruction of soft tissue by liquefactive necrosis, and decalcification of bone can occur. Treatment consists of 'neutralizing' the fluoride ion with calcium:
  —topically with 10% calcium gluconate gel
  —injection of the burn with calcium gluconate, repeated as necessary
  —infusing intra-arterial calcium gluconate or with Bier's type block.

Alkali

Alkalis are the commonest chemicals found in the home. They cause less immediate damage than acids but tend to have more long-term damage: saponification of fat and protein denaturation and progressive liquefactive necrosis that facilitates deeper penetration.

- **Sodium and potassium hydroxide.** These are the commonest chemicals in domestic use. They are present in many cleaning agents (oven cleaner, drain cleaner, bleach) and generate significant heat of dilution.
- **Cement.** The usual story is that the patient does not notice, or ignores, cement getting into their boots. Cement is caustic (pH 12–13), but acts slowly, and thus presentation tends to be delayed. Calcium oxide (lime) reacts with water (sweat) generating significant heat of dilution. It also reacts chemically to form calcium hydroxide (slaked lime) in an exothermic reaction.

Miscellaneous

- Hydrocarbons: some of these chemicals dissolve plasma membranes, causing superficial blistering. Systemic absorption of material may lead to respiratory depression.
- Phosphorus (found in insecticide and fertilizers): ignites on contact with water and so should be covered with oil. Irrigation with copper sulphate is a specific treatment.

Surgery

A major problem in the management of chemical burns is continued damage that results in deep wounds. Traditionally, one waited for demarcation to occur resulting in a deep lesion) before operating, as early excision and grafting often led to the unsatisfactory situation of skin grafts being damaged by residual chemicals. An alternative may be repeated shaving of the eschar until it is stable before grafting.

Extravasation injuries

These are not uncommon. Typically they occur on the dorsum of the hand or on the antecubital fossa, and can involve a variety of agents:

- hyperosmolar agents, e.g. contrast media, calcium gluconate, peripheral nutrition
- cytotoxic agents in those undergoing chemotherapy; damage is perpetuated by release of the chemical from dead cells. Injury can smoulder on for weeks
- vasopressor agents, often used in the ICU.

There is no consistency regarding cooling or warming of the injury:

- Cooling aims to limit spread by vasoconstriction but increases the toxicity of vinca alkaloids.
- Warming aims to dilute the chemical by vasodilatation but increases the toxicity of doxorubicin.

Others advocate infiltration of the area with hyalase in saline to disperse the chemical.
Surgical excision may be needed in some circumstances. Injuries in neonates tend to do surprisingly well.

Further reading

Kirkpatrick JJ, Enion DS, Burd DA. Hydrofluoric acid burns: a review. *Burns* 1995; **21**:483–93.

Cleft lip

Cleft lip (CL) is a defect of the primary palate resulting from the abnormal fusion of the maxillary and medial nasal processes. The lip is more commonly cleft on the left than on the right or bilaterally (6:3:1). Cleft lip, with or without an associated cleft palate (CL/P), is a different disease from the isolated cleft palate (CP), which is therefore described separately.

CL is commonest in Asians (0.2%), with twice the incidence in Caucasians (0.1%); it is uncommon in Afro-Caribbeans. There is a decreasing number of patients in developed countries due in part to a decrease in the birth rate but also to prenatal ultrasound diagnosis that leads to a variable rate of abortion, depending on cultural factors.

- CL/P is more common in males.
- If there is no family history, the risk is 1 in 100. If the father or one sibling has CL/P, then the risk is 4 in 100.
- CL/P may rarely occur as part of a syndrome: Patau (trisomy 13), Down's (trisomy 21).
- May be related to maternal phenytoin intake and smoking.
- Breast feeding may still be possible with CL.

Apart from a lip cleft of variable degree, there are other anatomical abnormalities:

- abnormal muscle attachment to the nose
- complex nasal deformity: cleft side is abnormal with deviated, dislocated cartilages and flattened nasal bones
- alveolar cleft at position of the canine
- shortened philtrum
- Simonart's band—a thin fibrous bridge over the upper lip cleft
- apart from the lip itself, the primary concerns are deformities of the alveolus/teeth and nose.

Treatment

It is important to prepare parents for multiple operations with an end point that may be difficult to define: the aim is to provide the opportunity for complete integration into society.

There are options with respect to:

- the timing of surgery
- the type of surgery.

Timing
Reconstructing the sphincter mechanism improves alveolar alignment, and so in theory it is preferable to perform surgery sooner rather than later. However, this is tempered with the need to perform surgery safely. **Traditionally**, the readiness for surgery was determined by the baby attaining the '10s', i.e., 10 pounds in weight, 10 weeks of age and a haemoglobin level of 10 g/dl. There is little firm evidence for optimal timing, but the overall trend has been for earlier surgery.

Fetal repair has been shown experimentally to be successful; there is no collagen scar, although there are also no skin appendages. However, it is not a clinical option due to the risk of inducing abortion.

Neonatal surgery remains a challenge. There is no definition of what constitutes 'neonatal', but it is generally taken to be 48h. There is supposed to be better healing and it may improve nasal development, as the tissue may still be malleable. There are supposed psychological benefits, and parents certainly prefer earlier repair. However, no significant overall advantage has been demonstrated. The baby's fitness for surgery is the main issue, and as neonates are obligate nasal breathers, there are additional concerns about the airway. Preparing for surgery by excluding concomitant disease and coordinating appropriate staff at short notice is a practical problem. In addition, the surgery is technically more difficult; consequently, only a minority of surgeons prefer this option.

Most surgeons will follow a **'conventional'** two-stage repair with:

- Repair of the lip and anterior palate at approximately 3 months (primary nose correction may also be performed). The previous view that early lip repair adversely affects nasal growth has not been proven.
- Repair of hard and soft palate at 6 months, with myringotomy with grommet insertion if required.

Delayed palatal repair is infrequently used in modern practice.

- These techniques aim to provide better mid-facial growth but at the expense of poor speech due to palatal incompetence.

Surgical techniques

Chinese surgeons were among the first to treat cleft lip by simply suturing the excised skin edges. Currently, there are many different techniques that use a variety of skin flaps to repair the upper lip. In general, all aim to reconstruct the continuity of the lip muscle after detachment from its abnormal insertions.

- **Millard rotation-advancement** is the most commonly used technique and is so-named because the cleft-side flap is advanced, whereas the non-cleft-side flap is rotated. The scar is well hidden along one border of the philtrum, except for the upper part. The advantages are that the pattern of incision lines is amenable to intraoperative adjustment, and revision surgery is possible; however, the learning curve is rather steep.
- **Tennison–Randall**, also known as the stencil method. The scar crosses the lower part of the philtrum, which can be flattened. The z-plasty achieves an attractive cupid's bow. Although the technique is easier to learn, it is difficult to adjust lip length intraoperatively if required.
- **Skoog.** Two triangular flaps from the lateral lip element are inset into the medial lip element to lengthen it.

Postoperative care

The aim is to protect the repairs:

- No bottle feeding for 5–10 days. Use syringes or special cups.

- Elbow splints.
- Breast feeding was traditionally discouraged on the grounds that it added extra strain, but more recent evidence suggests that the problem is overestimated and the risks are outweighed by the benefits of feeding.

Presurgical orthopaedics

Presurgical orthopaedics is an option that is regarded as useful by some, but its acceptance is not universal. It aims to narrow and correct alveolar alignment by passive or dynamic/active appliances, e.g. the Latham device, to facilitate surgery, reduce the need for bone grafts and improve final outcome. It is controversial as there are suggestions that it may actually be detrimental to growth. Some reserve it for use only in wide bilateral clefts. The use of lip adhesion is similarly controversial.

Other surgery to consider

- Pharyngoplasty for velopharyngeal incompetence.
- Bone grafting the alveolus to encourage eruption of teeth. This is usually delayed until after 9 years of age to reduce adverse effects on maxillary growth.

Further reading

Weinfeld AB, Hollier LH, Spira M, Stal S. International trends in the treatment of cleft lip and palate. *Clin Plast Surg* 2005; **32:**19–23.

Related topic of interest

- Cleft palate.

Cleft palate

Isolated cleft palate (CP) is a different disease from cleft lip, with or without a cleft palate (CL/P). Isolated CP is less common (30%) than CL/P and is more common in girls. There is little evidence of racial variations in incidence.

Embryology

The palatal shelves initially point vertically downward and after the tongue descends, they are able to rotate up, meet in midline and fuse. Any interference with this process causes defects or clefts in the secondary palate, posterior to the incisive foramen.
Clefts of the palate may be

- complete or incomplete
- unilateral or bilateral
- **submucous**—this condition is characterized by an uvula that is bifid to a variable degree, a palpable notch and a central 'blue line', indicating the separation of the palatal muscles. Twenty per cent of cases present with velopharyngeal incompetence (VPI).

Multifactorial environmental influences seem to be more important than genetic factors in CP: fetal alcohol syndrome, maternal smoking, anticonvulsant or retinoic acid therapy, and maternal diabetes have all been implicated. There is some evidence of folate deficiency being important, but the effect of folate supplements is inconclusive. Inheritance is weak; however, CP can sometimes occur in the context of a syndrome or in association with other abnormalities, e.g. Treacher–Collins syndrome, velocardiofacial syndrome (also called Shprintzen syndrome or DiGeorge syndrome, a defect in chromosome 22 leads also to thymic aplasia; psychological problems are seen in 10%), Aperts syndrome, Crouzon syndrome, Stickler syndrome and Pierre Robin sequence (hypoplastic mandible limits tongue descent that prevents rotation and subsequent fusion of the palatal shelves).

Classification

Kernahans Y classification, modified by Millard and Jackson, is a useful diagrammatic representation.
The Veau classification is descriptive:

- soft palate
- soft palate and hard palate
- soft palate and hard palate and unilateral prepalatal cleft
- soft palate and hard palate and bilateral prepalatal cleft.

Problems

- Speech
- Feeding. Babies with CP exhibit worse feeding than those with cleft lip, being

unable to generate a negative intra-oral pressure, but a trial of breast feeding is always worthwhile. A soft teat with an enlarged hole, with or without a squeezable bottle, can be used. Frequent burping is advised due to the excessive intake of air with feeding.
* Otitis media with hearing loss.
* Airway obstruction.

The aim of surgery is to close the palate to produce optimal speech whilst minimizing adverse effects on maxillary/midface growth. However, the balance is determined by the timing of surgery as well as by the surgical technique. Late surgery allows better midfacial growth but at the expense of speech development.

Timing

There has been great variation in timing in the past, but the general trend is toward early two-stage surgery—early anterior repair helps to narrow the hard palate cleft.

* repair of the lip and anterior palate 3/12; also primary nose correction
* repair of hard and soft palate 6/12, myringotomy with insertion of grommets.

It is generally advocated that repair of the palate should be complete by 18 months.

Surgical techniques

Repair of the hard palate
* **Veau–Kilner–Wardill technique**—also known as the 'push back' and probably the most common technique in current use. Large triangular mucosal flaps based on the greater palatine arteries are raised and rotated medially to meet in the midline. The donor bony surface is left uncovered and is usually packed with a haemostatic material such as Surgicel. New bone is formed under the periosteum. Fracture of the hamulus, which used to be part of this procedure, is no longer advocated.
* **Von Lagenbeck technique**—bipedicle flaps, based on and lateral to the great palatine arteries, are made by incising longitudinally, elevating and then suturing along the midline. The soft palate is not lengthened by this technique. Avoiding disturbance of the anterior palate reduces disturbances of growth centres and subsequent facial growth. There is a medial variant with narrower flaps that may allow better palatal growth but at the expense of a higher fistula rate due to the higher tension.
* For very narrow clefts, flapless repair may be performed, but as tissue is under some tension, postoperative fistulas are not uncommon.

Repair of the soft palate musculature
Repair involves detaching abnormal muscle insertions into the back of the hard palate and to reform the aponeurotic sling.

* intravelar veloplasty: muscle is freed, realigned and repaired in layers

• furlow with double opposing z-plasties. Lengthens the soft palate and results in better speech with less VPI.

Postoperative monitoring
Airway monitoring is important, particularly in Pierre Robin patients; obstruction may occur due to oedema, bleeding or secretions.

Complications
• fistula formation
• retarded maxillary growth, determined in part by the timing of the operation
• nasal obstruction.

Other treatments may be needed for the patient with cleft palate:

• speech therapy at 3–4 years
• pharyngoplasty at 5 years
• alveolar bone graft at 9 years or after
• orthodontics from 11 years onward.

Velopharyngeal incompetence

The inability to completely close off the gap between the soft palate and posterior pharyngeal wall allows air to escape, resulting in hypernasal speech. Velopharyngeal incompetence (VPI) is best assessed by:

• speech therapists
• fluoroscopy—allows real-time assessment of the problem
• nasoendoscopy—allows direct visualization.

Operative repair

Repair is required in approximately one-fifth of cases after surgery, although this rate is highly variable between different populations, which may reflect different cultural tolerances of speech defects. Pharyngoplasty procedures can be performed on the posterior or the lateral pharyngeal wall.

• Posterior wall augmentation with pharyngeal flaps (superiorly or inferiorly based); saturated to the soft palate and donor areas are left to heal by secondary intention. This provides a static repair.
• Lateral wall procedures (sphincter pharyngoplastics):
  —Hynes. A pair of superiorly based flaps (salpingopharyngeus) is elevated and rotated up to meet medially where they are sutured one above the other on the posterior wall to provide a bulky ridge. Donor areas are closed primarily.
  —Orticochea. Posterior tonsillar flaps (palatopharyngeus) are elevated, transposed medially and interdigitated into a small posterior pharyngeal flap. The donor areas heal by secondary intention and the scar helps with closure of the gap.

The procedure may lead to snoring, sleep apnoea or frank obstruction.

Further reading

Semb G, Brattstrom V, Molsted K et al. The Eurocleft study: intercenter study of treatment outcome in patients with complete cleft lip and palate: Part 1, Introduction and treatment experience. *Cleft Palate Craniofac J* 2005; **42:**64–8.

Related topics of interest

- Cleft lip
- Craniosynostosis.

Complications

A complication is the unintentional occurrence of an adverse medical condition that requires separate attention. Only a surgeon who does not operate can completely avoid complications.

The risk of surgical complications is increased in those with heart disease, lung disease and the obese. **Smokers** are at particularly high risk with an:

- increase in cardiac and pulmonary problems (even more than non-smokers with pre-existing heart or lung disease)
- increased flap necrosis
- increased wound infection
- increased rate of intensive care admissions and length of stay.

If the patient stops smoking for **at least** 6–8 weeks prior to surgery, the risk of mortality and morbidity can be significantly reduced.

Complications are typically classified by their **relationship to the operation itself**:

- general—those of a general nature, common to most operations
  —anaesthesia/sedation
  —trauma of surgery.
- specific—those limited to a specific operation. These will be discussed in the relevant chapters.

The **timing** can be either intraoperative, immediate (in the recovery room), early or late.

Anaesthetic complications

The risk of death due to a general anaesthetic alone (as opposed to the overall mortality after an operation) is commonly quoted in older studies as 1 in 10000, but this is an average for all surgery, including emergencies. It is probably nearer 1 in 200000–400000 for healthy patients undergoing elective surgery; the risk of complications is dependent upon concurrent illness, smoking, obesity and the surgery performed—long, complex or emergent.

- **Major complications** (approximately 1 in 1500)
  —**airway**—spasm, aspiration
  —**circulation**—excessive blood loss can cause hypovolaemia leading to arrhythmias, myocardial infarction and cerebrovascular accident. Deep vein thrombosis (DVT) and pulmonary embolism (PE) can also occur.
- Common minor side effects include sore throat, nausea, vomiting and delayed recovery.

Malignant hyperthermia is a rare, life-threatening complication of general anaesthesia that requires both:

- **genetic predisposition** in the form of (heterogenetic autosomal dominant trait that occurs in about 1 in 10000), and

- **triggering agents** (typically volatile anaesthetics and depolarizing muscle relaxants). The mechanism is unclear but abnormal calcium handling is suggested.

Malignant hyperthermia is a hypermetabolic crisis that causes contraction of skeletal muscle and can be extremely dangerous:

- rigidity, e.g. masseter (early sign)
- increased energy consumption with hypercarbia and metabolic acidosis (early sign), increased serum potassium and creatine kinase and myoglobinuria from plasma membrane damage
- tachycardia and arrhythmias
- rhabdomyolysis can be used as an indicator of severity
- **increased temperature is actually a late sign**.

Specific treatment is dantrolene; other management includes 100% oxygen. Stop the trigger and use alternatives; depending on the severity of the problem, surgery may be allowed to proceed.

Wound infection

In terms of infection risk, surgical wounds are usually classified as in Table 1.

Most elective plastic surgery operations are considered **clean**, and prophylactic antibiotics are of doubtful benefit, with the additional risk of promoting the development of multi-drug resistance. However, when implants or other foreign bodies are involved and infection is a potentially serious complication, prophylactic antibiotics are warranted to be of practical use, the antibiotic needs to be administered such that therapeutic doses are attained at the time of the first incision and are maintained for the duration of the operation and for a few hours afterwards. Usually no more than three doses are given for prophylaxis.

Certain factors predispose to wound infection:

- general—age, malnutrition, obesity, immunosuppression
- local—necrotic tissue, ischaemia, foreign bodies and haematomas
- micro-organisms—virulence, load and antibiotic resistance.

Table 1 Infection risk of different types of surgical wound.

Type	Details	Infection risk
Clean	No viscus opened, e.g. most plastic surgery operations	<2%
Clean–contaminated	Viscus opened without spillage of contents, e.g. operations involving the oropharynx, i.e. head and neck cancer operations	<10%
Contaminated	Viscus with spillage of contents or inflammation	<20%
Dirty	Abscess formation or visceral perforation, retained necrotic tissue	~40%

> Surgical site infections (SSI)—superficial and deep incisional, organ/space infections
>
> To qualify as a superficial incisional infection the problem must:
>
> - occur within 30 days of surgery
> - involves only the skin and subcutaneous tissue with at least one of the following: pain/tenderness, redness/heat or swelling
> - either purulent discharge or organisms cultured.

Principles of management include:

- microbiological confirmation—culture and sensitivity, gram stain
- treatment—drain any collections, broad spectrum antibiotics can be administered while waiting for results. The incision wound may have to be laid open and closed after a delay.

Haemorrhage

Bleeding is increased in patients taking aspirin and warfarin or in those with excessive alcohol consumption; some herbal remedies are also implicated. It is important to elicit a specific, full and precise drug history, as the patient may not regard some of these as 'drugs'. All such drugs should be stopped prior to elective surgery wherever possible. Bleeding can be categorized according to the timing:

- primary—during surgery
- reactive—immediately postoperative, usually as a result of raised blood pressure
- secondary—often due to infection.

Minor bleeding may be managed with pressure/packing; more severe bleeding may need formal haemostasis with diathermy, ties or clipping.

Haematoma

Haematomas will liquefy after approximately 10 days, and eventually organize to leave an area of fibrous scarring, but may become infected in the meantime.

- Minor haematomas can be left or incised and drained early to avoid infection/scarring.
- Large haematomas generally require formal evacuation; problems may also arise due to the volume of blood lost and flap necrosis may result from the pressure effect.
  —Serial aspiration with pressure dressings may work, but often is unsuccessful due to clots; in addition pressure dressings will obscure the wound.
  —Antibiotics are probably prudent as there is a risk of infection, but their usefulness has not been properly examined.

Pyrexia

Pyrexia after an operation is not uncommon; the timing provides important clues to the underlying reason (see Table 2). A useful way to remember the common causes are the 'W's: **wind** (pulmonary), **water** (urinary tract), **wound**, **walk** (DVT) and **'wonder drugs'**.

Hypoxia ('desaturation')

Hypoxia occurs in 10% of postoperative patients and is associated with increased morbidity and mortality. It may present with reduced consciousness or changes in emotion or perception.

It may be caused by:

- poor ventilation, e.g. airway obstruction, bronchospasm, shunting (atelectasis), opiates or **aspiration**
- poor lung perfusion causing ventilation perfusion mismatch, e.g. pulmonary embolism, or poor cardiac output, e.g. **arrhythmias**
- reduced diffusion across the alveolar membrane due to pneumonia or pulmonary oedema.

Table 2   The causes and features of pyrexia.

Timing	Likely causes	Features
First day	Systemic response to the tissue damage of surgery, but also possibly: • haematomas • pre-existing infection.	Typically low grade (<38°C)
Day 1–3	Atelectasis (48h) or chest infection (later)	Atelectasis (minor lung collapse) is common, particularly after abdominal operations. Patients present with pyrexia, tachypnoea and tachycardia. Thick and copious secretions cause airway collapse and reduced tidal volume. It is more frequent in smokers, the overweight and those with pre-existing lung disease. It is generally treated with intensive chest physiotherapy; antibiotics and nebulizers are needed sometimes
Day 3–7	Chest infection, wound infection or urinary tract infection	Dyspnoea, cough and some chest pain. Localizing signs and symptoms for wound or urinary infection
Day 7–10	DVT/PE	Calf pain, swelling and tenderness Dyspnoea, tachycardia and haemoptysis

Aspiration risk is increased in the obese, the pregnant, those with pre-existing gastrointestinal disease or with inadequate fasting. The aspirated stomach contents cause chemical pneumonitis that may become secondarily infected, particularly with anaerobic or gram-negative micro-organisms. The apical part of the right lower lobe is most frequently involved as it is the most dependent segment when supine.

- If noticed early, the pharynx may be suctioned out with the head tilted down.
- Prophylactic antibiotics may reduce the chance of secondary infection.
- Steroids have not been shown to reduce inflammation.

Arrhythmias may reflect abnormalities such as cardiac ischaemia or pulmonary embolism. It can sometimes also be caused by the anaesthesia (general or local) or by metabolic disturbances such as hypoxia, hypercapnia, electrolyte disturbance and acidosis as well as hypovolaemia. Management includes finding the cause and treating it.

Laser complications

Lasers are sources of high energy and precautions are needed to avoid the hazards.

- **Eye damage.** Laser light can lead to permanent eye damage—CO_2 wavelengths damage the lens and cornea, whereas visible light wavelengths damage the retinal vasculature and pigments. Protective eyewear is needed and reflective surfaces in the treatment room should be avoided.
- **Laser plume** (smoke). CO_2 lasers create smoke and Q-switched lasers produce a splatter. Plume smoke has been shown to contain viable particles: human papilloma virus (HPV) has been cultured from the smoke after wart treatment. Smoke evacuators, gloves and high-filtration masks are recommended.

Lasers may cause hyperpigmentation, hypopigmentation, crusting, scarring, blistering and wound infections. Scarring used to be a dreaded complication of skin resurfacing with continuous-wave CO_2 lasers, but is less common with modern pulsed lasers. Complications may be reduced by the careful adjusting of the parameters, but cannot be avoided totally.

- **Ablative lasers for skin resurfacing, e.g. CO_2**—hyperpigmentation and erythema may last for months; delayed hypopigmentation, milia, acne, herpes reactivation, and hypertrophic scarring are possible.
- **Hair removal with long-pulsed lasers**—hyperpigmentation (especially if tanned or dark skinned), temporary hypopigmentation in 10%.
- **Vascular lasers, e.g. pulsed dye lasers (PDL)**—purpura lasting 1–2 weeks.
- **Tattoo and pigmented lesion removal (Q-switched lasers)**—blistering, crusting (can be reduced with cooling techniques) and hypopigmentation, particularly after multiple treatments in darker-skinned patients. Some flesh-coloured tattoos with ferric oxide may become darker after conversion by laser energy to the ferrous form; anaphylactic reactions have been reported in a minority of patients. This may be due to the laser causing 're-exposure' or altering the tattoo pigment antigenicity.

Further reading

Moller A, Villebro N, Pedersen T, Tonnensen H. Effect of preoperative smoking intervention on postoperative complications: a randomized clinical trial. *Lancet* 2002; **359**:114–17.

Related topics of interest

- Hair removal
- Keloids and hypertrophic scarring
- Lasers: principles
- Tattoo removal
- Vascular anomalies.

Craniosynostosis

Craniosynostosis is the premature fusion of the fibrous joints of skull sutures. This may happen to any of the sutures leading to distinctive abnormalities of skull shape as growth perpendicular to the suture line is retarded (Virchow's Law), although this is an oversimplification of the compensatory growth pattern.

- Simple craniosynostosis affects one suture.
- Complex craniosynostosis affects two or more sutures.
- Syndromic craniosynostosis is associated with other abnormalities and is usually complex.

The brain triples in size in the first year, and bony restriction of expansion may lead to raised intracranial pressure (ICP): with a single suture synostosis, ICP is raised in 13%; with multiple sutures, it is raised in 40%. Hydrocephalus is more common in syndromic cases and may further increase ICP.

Radiologically there is loss of the usual lucency and suture interdigitations with increased sclerosis. If the ICP is raised for a long time, the flat bones may have a 'copper-beaten' or 'thumb printing' appearance. The various sutures that can be involved in craniosynostosis are shown in Table 1.

Craniosynostosis can occur in isolation (related to toxic/gestational influences) or syndromic (especially coronal). The commonest syndromes associated with craniosynostosis are Crouzon's syndrome and Apert's syndrome.

Crouzon's syndrome

This is characterized by:

- Skull abnormalities. The commonest abnormality is a flattened skull (turribrachycephaly) due to bicoronal synostosis, but other sutures can be involved. These patients may also have hydrocephalus, contributing further to raised ICP (>20 mmHg unstressed) that is manifested by bulging fontanelles, irritability or fits, papilloedema (pathognomonic feature) and optic atrophy. Nystagmus and strabismus are associated features.
- Midfacial hypoplasia. There is a wide range of severity. A class III bite (prognathic) is common.
- Recurrent middle-ear infections and conductive hearing loss.

These features are also found in Apert's syndrome, but in Crouzon's, the midfacial hypoplasia tends to be uniformly more severe, and shallow orbits can lead to rather profound proptosis. Mental retardation is not a common feature (5%).

- Hands are normal
- Cleft palate is unusual.

Apert's syndrome

Apert's is one of the acrocephalosyndactyly syndromes (i.e. inherited disorder affecting skull, face, hands and feet. Most cases are sporadic (possibly related to increasing

Table 1 Features of craniosynostosis involving various sutures.

Suture involved	Deformity	Notes
Plagiocephaly (Greek for oblique)	Coronal (anterior) or lambdoid (posterior, less common)	Majority of plagiocephaly seen is 'deformational' or 'positional' to distinguish from 'true' plagiocephaly due to a synostosis. Its occurrence is increasing due to the tendency to nurse babies supine to reduce 'cot-death'. In true plagiocephaly, it may be associated with torticollis, prematurity, oligohydramnios or other causes of uterine constraint. Harlequin orbits may lead to ulceration and blindness due to severe proptosis.
Trigonocephaly (triangular)	Metopic	Less than 10% are syndromic. Often with hypotelorism. Usually resolves with time
Scaphocephaly (narrow and long)	Sagittal	Commonest synostosis (more than half). Usually sporadic. Males more frequently affected
Brachycephaly	Bilateral coronal	Commonly syndromic. Short skull with compensatory growth superiorly if untreated, leading to a tower-like appearance, hence 'turribrachycephaly'

paternal age), but some are inherited in an autosomal dominant manner. It shares many similarities with Crouzon's syndrome, but also has

- syndactyly that is usually complex
- cleft palate in 20%
- small beaked nose, anti-mongoloid slant, hypertelorism
- acne/hyperhidrosis.

Mental retardation can occur in the absence of a raised ICP due to hydrocephalus or other brain abnormalities such as agenesis of the corpus callosum.

Other craniosynostosis syndromes include:

- Pfeiffer (also includes hand abnormalities)
- Carpenter
- Saethre-Chotzen (these three are examples of acrocephalosyndactyly).

Most syndromes are autosomal dominant (except Carpenter's, which is recessive) with variable penetrance and are associated with mutations in fibroblastic growth factor (FGF) receptor genes.

Treatment

Treatment is prolonged and multi-staged.
   The priorities are rather simple:

- Correct breathing problems. This may be as simple as a tonsillectomy, but may require a formal skeletal advancement or gradual distraction. Tracheostomy may be necessary.
- Protect the brain. Relieve ICP quickly: ICP is inversely related to intellectual development.
- Protect the eyes.
- Optimize feeding. Nutrition should be adequate. Dental hygiene is important.

Sorting out these basic priorities will allow the patient to be in optimal shape for subsequent treatment:

- Craniectomy—at 3 months of age or earlier if the ICP is too high. Bony gaps are easily reconstituted in those less than 2 years of age.
- Frontofacial advancement within a year.
- Maxillary/midface advancement (Le Fort advancement or gradual distraction) at 9–12 years of age.

Further reading

Cohen SR, Persing JA. Intracranial pressure in single suture synostosis. *Cleft Palate Craniofac J* 1998; **35:**194–6.

Related topic of interest

- Cleft palate.

Dupuytren's disease

Dupuytren's disease (DD) is a benign but chronic and progressive disease characterized by the proliferation of contractile fibroblastic cells involving the palmar fascia, with knuckle pads (Garrods), palm nodules and cord contractures of the fingers. Guillaume Dupuytren was Napoleon's surgeon; the condition had been previously described by others including Astley-Cooper.

DD is bilateral in around two-thirds of cases but affects the right hand more frequently. The ring finger is most frequently involved with the little and middle fingers next. The disease may cause various problems:

- Functional problems occur when the bent fingers hinder work or simple activities, e.g. they may catch on the sides of pockets.
- Cosmetic.
- Some mild to moderate discomfort may occur with the disease; severely contracted fingers may dig into the palm.

DD is usually described as being more common in those of Celtic origin. It affects 3% of the US population and is less common in Afro-Caribbeans and Asians; Orientals tend to have palmar disease without finger contractures. It affects men much more frequently, peaking at 50 years of age (earlier than in women).

There is some evidence to suggest that microscopic inflammation is an important part of the pathogenesis of the disease. Hypoxia and free radicals may stimulate fibroblasts; biochemically, the entire fascia is abnormal even if not clinically affected (altered metalloproteinase activity, increased collagen III and growth factor sensitivity). Secondary changes may occur; the digital neurovascular bundle is shifted toward the midline, especially if the proximal interphalangeal joint (PIPJ) is affected, or the extensor central slip is stretched by fibrotic transverse retinacular ligament leading to a boutonniere type deformity.

DD may afflict other sites, e.g. the sole (Ledderhose—plantar fibromatosis) and the penis (Peyronies)—patients with involvement of all three sites are deemed to have **Dupuytren's diathesis**. They tend to have a particularly aggressive form of the disease with a higher chance of recurrence after surgery. Such patients may also have an association with retroperitoneal fibrosis. These patients are generally younger and have a strong family history.

Risk factors

The exact cause is unknown but there are many associations:

- Some families show autosomal dominant type inheritance with variable penetrance. The gene has not yet been found.
- Physical: posttraumatic, especially Colle's fracture; vibration white finger doubles the risk.
- Metabolic
  —Diabetics have a 5–10 times increased risk that is related to duration of disease and presence of retinopathy rather than severity per se. The disease tends to be less severe and the radial digits are more likely to be affected.

—Thyroid disease: both over- and underactivity, but particularly hypothyroid.
—Hyperlipidaemia.
- Associations with alcohol and alcoholic liver disease are not clear cut and associations with epilepsy could be due to either the treatment or the disease itself.

Staging

The severity of disease is staged according to the sum of the contracture at the PIPJ and MCP joints (Tubiana): 0–45° stage 1, 49–90° stage 2, 90–135° stage 3 and 135–180° stage 4.

The table top test is an empirical test with the palm placed flat on a table top: in moderate disease, the patient cannot lift the finger off the table, but in more severe cases, the fingers cannot even straighten to lie flat.

Treatment

Medical treatment

Splintage and physiotherapy is generally considered not to be effective as a treatment but can be used preoperatively. Preoperative stretching (continuous elongation technique) is of unproven benefit. Radiotherapy is certainly no longer recommended.

- There are a wide variety of other proposed treatments:
  —Some are of possible benefit but are unproven to date: colchicines, allopurinol, tamoxifen, 5FU, interferon alpha 2b, interferon gamma and calcium channel blockers (verapamil).
  —Others are probably of little benefit: ultrasound, vitamin E.
- Cortisone injection may soften and slow disease in knuckle pads and nodules, but has little effect on cords.
- Clostridium collagenase (Cordase) injections are currently entering a phase III FDA trial, but do seem to involve high recurrence rates.
  —Connective tissue growth factor blocking antibodies are entering phase I trials.

Surgery

The following are the common recommendations for considering surgical treatment:

- metacarpophalangeal (MCPJ) joint contracture of more than 30°
- PIPJ contracture of any degree
- contracture of the first web space, causing thumb adduction
- painful nodules or pads.
- Closed cord rupture has been reported anecdotally, usually related to accidental trauma, and is not recommended as a therapeutic option.
- Fasciotomy (open) is suitable for minimal disease.
- Fasciectomy is used for more severe disease. Total radical fasciectomy produces similar results to regional fasciectomy but with more complications—swelling and stiffness.
- Dermafasciectomy is recommended for recurrent or aggressive disease (particularly in those with a diathesis) or when the skin is involved. The concept of a 'firebreak graft' placed at flexion creases comes from the observation that there are fewer recurrence tendencies under skin grafts.

Needle aponeurotomy (NA), also known as needle fasciotomy, is gaining acceptance outside of France, where it originated many years ago. A percutaneous fasciotomy can performed as an outpatient technique under local anaesthesia. A needle bevel is used to slowly saw through the band (previously a blade was used) and until recently, showed little acceptance outside of France. NICE approval in the UK was gained in 2004.

Recurrence is inevitable whatever the treatment, therefore safety should be an important consideration, as well as efficacy. The results of NA approach those of open surgery (>50% recurrence at 5 years) and whilst the results are not as long lasting, the procedure can be safely repeated as required. Recovery is quicker and patient satisfaction higher, but this has not been objectively compared. NA is suited to treatment of early-stage disease and is particularly recommended for the elderly. It is not suitable for diffuse or severe disease, cases with tethered skin, MCPJ contracture or previous open surgery. Approximately 10–15% of cases need open surgery rather than NA. Complication rates of less than 1% are quoted and include skin breaks, nerve injury, tendon injury and infection.

Results of surgery overall:

- Worse outcome with early onset disease, severe PIPJ contracture and little-finger involvement.
- With worse disease, surgery is less likely to provide full correction.
- Best/most predictable results are achieved in MCPJ contractures.
- PIPJ disease, especially of the little finger, is most likely to have recurrent problems (50% on average).

Complications of surgery:

- infection
- recurrence 40–75% after 5 years, more likely if little finger (especially PIPJ) is involved, young age of onset, diathesis
- nerve injuries 17–41%, doubled with surgery for recurrences
- flare reaction is more common in women
- stiffness.

Further reading

Foucher G, Medina J, Navarro R. Percutaneous needle aponeurotomy: complications and results. *J Hand Surg (Br)* 2003; **28:**427–31.

Ear reconstruction

Ear reconstruction may be required when there is:

- congenital malformation, e.g. microtia (children)
- acquired loss: after trauma or extirpation of cancer (adults).

Microtia

This condition occurs in 1 in 7000 Caucasians, and is slightly more common in Asians.

- bilateral or unilateral
- almost twice as common on the right (right:left:bilateral 5:3:1)
- males are affected three times more frequently than females.

Generally, the cause is unknown; some cases demonstrate patterns suggestive of multifactorial inheritances and there have been reported associations with maternal rubella and thalidomide exposure. One-third of cases have other associated abnormalities: often with first and second arch underdevelopment. Ten per cent of these are part of defined syndromes such as Treacher–Collins or Goldenhar syndrome.

There can be a wide spectrum of deformity. The ear may be no more than a rudimentary skin appendage.

- **Lobular**—a sausage-shaped mass consists mostly of the lobule remnant. The external ear canal is often absent.
- **Conchal**—more earlike in appearance and the ear canal is variably present. This is a less common variant.
- The hairline is often low on the abnormal side

Microtia can be graded:

- grade 1: small but normal
- grade 2: small but missing features
- grade 3: rudimentary lobule and cartilage
- grade 4: complete anotia.

There are two main options for these patients with respect to the external ear:

- reconstruction
- prosthetic ear.

Local preferences are a strong determining factor in the choice of technique. Autogenous reconstruction is the treatment of choice in many countries, including the USA, but prosthetics are the main choice in Sweden (home of the Branemark prosthesis).

Reconstruction

To reconstruct an ear, there is a need to find cartilage or its equivalent to make a framework, and then have skin to cover it. There is a choice of material available for the framework.

- Silicone scaffolds are prone to extrusion, but results with porous polyethylene (Medpor, Porex) are more encouraging, although long-term results are yet unknown.
- Allograft/xenograft—these materials suffer from absorption; there is a small risk of transmitting infection.
- Autogenous material:
  —Costal cartilage—the most popular choice
  —contralateral ear and ear remnant—rarely used.

Timing of surgery

At the age of 5 years, the normal ear is >85% of adult size and can be used as a reference. The reconstructed ear continues to grow, albeit at a reduced pace. The other major determinant of timing is waiting for the costal cartilage to be large enough to take a graft from; this is usually achieved when the child is about 6 years old. There has been a tendency to wait longer, from 7 to 10 years old, depending on the exact technique.

The surgery consists of a variable number of stages depending on the exact technique: the 'classical' Tanzer techniques is three-staged. Alternatives include the Brent and the Nagata techniques. The choice of technique depends in part on the size of the ear that is present. The ear is often left for at least six months between stages to allow the blood supply to be re-established.

- **First stage.** A costal cartilage framework is made and put into position. A template, usually made out of underdeveloped X-ray film, can be used to assist in this process; careful planning is vital. An ear shape is carved out from the sixth to eighth costal cartilages and held together either with sutures or wires. A pocket at the proposed position is dissected out for this; excessive dissection should be avoided to prevent subsequent displacement of the cartilage. Mattress sutures are used to improve definition of the ear contours, with or without bolsters. A suction drain is placed, and an ear bandage worn for 7–10 days.
- **Second stage.** The ear scaffold is elevated from the side of the head. This exposes a bare postauricular sulcus—part of the elevated skin will drape over the cartilage rim while the remainder is covered with fascia (temporoparietal or post-auricular) and a skin graft—either a full-thickness graft from the groin or a split-thickness graft from thigh. There may be reconstruction of the lobule and tragus, depending on the exact technique.
- **Third stage.** Definitive reconstruction of the tragus and lobule.

Nagata transfers the lobule in the first stage, as well as reconstructing the tragus and posterior wall of the concha; his two-stage technique is performed at 10 years of age when the cartilage is said to provide a sturdier framework for more detailed carving and a better result.

Hearing restoration surgery can be performed by ENT surgeons between stages if necessary.

Specific complications after surgery include:

- infection
- loss of skin graft or cartilage
- pneumothorax from harvesting costal cartilage is rare.

Ear prosthesis

Originally, silicone prostheses were fixed with adhesives that could be quite messy; the Branemark (1995) technique using osseointegration (titanium anchor in the temporal bone) was a major development. The common indications for preferring prosthesis over autogenous reconstruction are:

- Failed autogenous reconstruction: previous scarring hinders surgery and so may need temporoparietal or free flaps to provide vascularized tissue. There may also be reluctance on the part of the patient to have another operation.
- Hypoplastic soft tissue/skeleton.
- Low hairline—this would leave a hairy upper pole but it is not an insurmountable problem as one can use standard hair removal techniques. It is actually the lower pole and overall positioning that is much more important for cosmesis.
- Acquired defects, especially with an intact tragus that can disguise the anterior margin of the prosthesis.

However, for prostheses:

- Meticulous hygiene is required.
- The patient has the constant reminder of a false ear.
- The materials degrade and require changing every 2–5 years.
- The anterior margin is difficult to disguise.
- The overall cost is actually higher.

Further reading

Nagata S. A new method of total reconstruction of the auricle for microtia. *Plast Reconstr Surg* 1993; **92:**187–201.

Related topics of interest

- Craniosynostosis
- Hair removal.

Electrical burns

Electricity can cause injuries with thermal and non-thermal components:

- **Thermal**—the skin resistance to the flow of electrical current will cause heat generation (Joule effect) resulting in charring at the contact points (also called the entry and exit points). Electrical current flowing through a limb will cause heating of bone because of its low resistance, and being deep in the limb, the heat does not dissipate easily.
  —Clothing may be ignited causing a flame burn.
- **Non-thermal**—massive depolarization damages excitable tissue such as:
  —Cardiac conducting system resulting in cardiac arrest due to ventricular fibrillation (VF) or other arrhythmias.
  —Brain tissue, causing loss of consciousness. Involvement of the respiratory centre in the medulla can cause respiratory arrest.

It is conventional to categorize electrical burns according to the magnitude of the voltage involved.

Low voltage (less than 1000 V)

This is the commonest type of electrical injury and occurs mostly in the home. Young children are often involved as their natural inquisitiveness leads them to explore their environment—chewing on electrical flex or inserting their fingers or objects into electrical sockets; as a result, injuries usually involve the hands or mouth. Depending on the characteristics of the current, there may be tetany; the patient may be unable to let go and the strong muscular contractions may cause fractures or dislocations. The cutaneous injury may be similar to thermal burns.

High voltage (more than 1000 V)

Higher voltages may causes deep and often extensive muscle injury (with deceptively little damage of overlying skin), with rhabdomyolysis and myoglobinuria that may lead to blockage of the renal tubules and renal failure. Muscle damage may be indicated by:

- hyperkalaemia
- acidosis
- raised creatinine and creatine phosphokinase
- myoglobin in the blood.

It is important to be watchful for **compartment syndrome**. Clinical assessment is less reliable as the nerve symptoms due to direct electrical damage may be indistinguishable from compartment syndrome. Compartment pressure monitoring should be used if available. Tissue damage without significant temperature change is said to occur by 'electroporation'; the current disrupts the lipid membrane forming pores that increase passive permeability. MRI demonstrates muscle necrosis very well and radionuclide scanning may be oversensitive; however, the availability of these may be limited.

The patient may be thrown by the force, causing fractures/dislocation. Arcing may cause very high temperatures resulting in full-thickness wounds; the exit wound tends to be bigger.

Arrhythmias, especially ectopics, right bundle branch block and supraventricular tachycardia, are found in a third of high-voltage injuries. The risk of VF actually decreases with very high currents. The passage of current from hand to hand is associated with much higher mortality compared with hand-to-foot passage.

Ultra high voltage, e.g. lightning

The energy level is very high but is of very short duration. Injuries may be due to a direct strike (with typically high mortality) or a 'side flash' due to discharge of current through the ground or air near a structure that has been struck by lightning.

- Brief loss of consciousness, weakness or paraesthesia is common.
- Cardiorespiratory arrest may require **prolonged** resuscitation.
- Fractures, and injuries of the eye and ear may result; tympanic membrane perforation is one of the commonest reported complications.

Lichtenberg figures are an arborescent pattern on the skin that is pathognomonic of lightning strike, and generally disappear within 24h.

If the patient survives, there may be chronic sequelae such as:

- cataracts
- neurological problems—epilepsy, peripheral nerve demyelination, spinal cord problems.

Management

Remove the patient safely from cause—10000V can jump several centimetres.

- **Airway.** Cervical spine may be damaged by intense contractions or a fall. It is vital to maintain cervical stability while keeping the airway open.
- **Breathing.** Electrical effects on the medulla may cause respiratory arrest.
- **Circulation.** Gross cardiac damage is relatively rare but may cause cardiac arrest or arrhythmias. Prolonged cardiopulmonary resuscitation may be needed.

The secondary survey is a head-to-toe inspection: in particular, check for:

- entry/exit wounds
- cutaneous burns
- nerve dysfunction.

An ECG is required on admission in all electrical injuries; continuous monitoring for 24h is advised in those who suffered a cardiac arrest and in those who may have had current passing through the heart (hand-to-hand current passage).

Resuscitation should be aimed at both the thermal and electrical components. Any muscle necrosis will raise the fluid requirement; titrate crystalloid resuscitation to the urine output rather than the burn surface area, which may be deceptively small. A rate of 1–1.5 ml/kg/h is reasonable. Myoglobinuria requires aggressive resuscitation and urine alkalinization using bicarbonate.

Debridement of any non-viable skin and muscle follows general surgical principles; the muscle necrosis after an electrical burn is recognized to be non-progressive, contrary to earlier opinions. There is no general agreement with regard the timing of surgery; some advocate early surgery to reduce the time of inflammation and wound repair, while others wait for the full extent of tissue damage to become apparent.

Further reading

Rai J, Jeschke MG, Barrow RE, Herndon DN. Electrical injuries: a 30-year review. *J Trauma* 1999; **46:**933–6.

Related topic of interest

• Acute burns.

Extensor tendon injuries

The repair of extensor tendon injuries of the hand is often delegated to junior surgeons. If extensor injuries are not dealt with appropriately, they can lead to significant loss of flexion and extension from adhesions and from excessive tendon shortening or lengthening. The general points about tendon nutrition and tendon healing are discussed in another chapter (Flexor tendon injuries).

Anatomy

The extensor digitorum communis arises from the common extensor origin on the lateral epicondyle of the humerus. Tendons arise and pass along the forearm and under the extensor retinaculum into the dorsum of the hand. The hood-like extensor expansion covers the dorsal aspect of the middle and proximal phalanges; the central slip inserts into the base of the middle phalanx, and the terminal extensor tendon formed by the convergence of the lateral bands inserts into the base of the distal phalanx.

The extensor tendons are divided into several zones, as shown in Table 1.

In general, injuries in odd-numbered zones are more difficult to treat because they overlie joints (zones 1, 3 and 5) or involve multiple tendons (zone 7).

Management

Common injuries include:

- open trauma—lacerations and fight/punch injuries
- closed injuries may occur with forceful flexion of the extended joint or through crush injuries
- attrition—rheumatoid arthritis at the wrist level, especially on the ulnar side
- tendon laceration results in extensor lag with reduced active extension of the MCPS against resistance. It is important to actively exclude other injuries such as nerves and bones.

Table 1 Description of extensor tendon zones.

Extensor zone	Description
1	Over the distal interphalangeal joint (DIPJ)
2	Between the proximal interphalangeal joint (PIPJ) and the DIPJ
3	Over the PIPJ
4	Between the metacarpophalangeal joint (MCPJ) and the PIPJ
5	Over the MCPJ
6	Between the MCPJ and the extensor retinaculum (ER)
7	Over the ER
8	Between the ER and the musculotendinous junction

Passive and active movements at each joint should be systematically tested. X-rays may be useful to diagnose associated fractures.

- Tendon repair should be performed preferably within 6 h, but 12 h is acceptable if antibiotics are administered. Infected tooth puncture injuries should preferably be closed after a delay when infection and swelling has resolved.
- Exposure of extensor tendons is easier than for flexor tendons.
- There is no general agreement regarding mode of repair. Repair strength is related to the number of sutures crossing the break; it is important to avoid bunching and causing tendon shortening that will compromise the function of the digit.
  —continuous horizontal mattress or 'figure of eight'—easy, quick and minimal shortening
  —the modified Bunnell or Kessler is stronger and in common use
  —MGH (Massachusetts General Hospital) repair (4 strands) with crossing running suture is more resistant to gaping. Particularly recommended for zone 6, where early mobilization may be preferential.
- Some have a preference for absorbable sutures over monofilament synthetics because they are supposed to extrude less.
- Partial lacerations that are proximal to the MCPJ may not require repair.

Specific injuries

Distal interphalangeal joint (DIPJ), zone 1

Division of the conjoint tendon at this level will result in reduced extension—a mallet finger deformity—that may eventually cause a swan neck deformity due to tendon imbalance. Significant functional impairment with pain and stiffness may result if it is left untreated.

Open injury (type II mallet): carry out primary tendon repair if possible; however, the tendon is flat and ribbon-like and may be difficult to suture satisfactorily. Postoperative splintage for 6 weeks with 2 weeks of night splintage is needed; some prefer pin fixation of the DIPJ to maintain a degree of hyperextension.

Closed injury (type I mallet):

- If there is no bone involvement, then a mallet splint can be used to maintain hyperextension (avoid skin blanching) for 6 weeks followed by 2 weeks of night splinting, and then active extension after 8 weeks. This option requires a high level of patient compliance; the patient must understand that extension needs to be *continuous*.
- If there is a small fracture, closed reduction may still be suitable. K wires can be used to provide fixation for 6 weeks, followed by splintage for 2 weeks after its removal; there is a small risk of osteomyelitis.
- In a small number, there may be a fracture that is large or rotated; in such cases, accurate reduction is needed. This usually requires open reduction and fixation, although it can be difficult and is associated with a rather high complication rate such as joint stiffness or avascular necrosis of the fracture fragment. Alternatives include extension block K wiring or using miniature external fixators.

Persistent mallet deformity can be treated:

- further splintage (worthwhile up to several months)

- resection of a more proximal tendon segment
- arthrodesis of DIPJ with 100° flexion.

Proximal interphalangeal joint (PIPJ), zone 3

Injuries in this region will lead to a 'boutonniere' deformity due to button-holing of the head of the middle phalanx through the disrupted central slip of the extensor expansion.

- **Open injury**—lacerations over the PIPJ mean a central slip rupture until proven otherwise. The tendon is repaired with the joint in full extension and then splinted.
- **Closed injury**—selected injuries can be treated by splintage or K wire, particularly in the uncooperative. Involvement of a large bony fragment requires open treatment.

Metacarpophalangeal joint (MCPJ), zone 5

Commonly, a fight injury; the tooth lacerates the tendon and contaminates the joint; the middle and ring finger are most frequently involved. There is often a delay in presentation because of intoxication at the time of injury; the injury is potentially very serious as it can lead to amputation if neglected.

- broad-spectrum intravenous antibiotics
- primary tendon repair can be considered if there is no evidence of clinical infection
- delayed repair of tendon if there is any infection.

Postoperatively, the fingers should be splinted in comfortable full extension for 3 weeks with the interphalangeal joints free and with more extension in middle and ring fingers.

Rehabilitation

The exact program depends on the level of injury and preferences of the surgeon. It takes about 12 weeks to recover to full strength; most regimes involve protective mobilization:

- **Injuries distal to MCPJ**—(mallet, boutonniere) the DIPJ and PIPJ are immobilized in extension for approximately 4–6 weeks.
- **Injuries proximal to MCPJ**—maintain MCPJ extension for 2–4 weeks, then splint in a position that allows active flexion and passive extension. The PIPJ should be left free to move.

Light (clerical) work at 6 weeks, medium work at 8 weeks and heavy work at 10 weeks. The patient can drive (6 weeks), with any contact sport delayed until after 12 weeks.

Complications

- Commonest complication is adhesion, causing stiffness and loss of flexion and extension —it is more likely if there has been trauma to tendon (including iatrogenic injury) —immobilization.

- Loss of flexion due to shortening of extensor tendon or adhesions
- Extrinsic and intrinsic tendon tightness often follows crush injuries
- Rupture of tendon
- Dorsal skin necrosis from inappropriate splintage
- Infection.

Further reading

Newport ML, Williams CD. Biomechanical characteristics of extensor suture techniques. *J Hand Surg (US)* 1992; **17:**1117–23.

Related topic of interest

- Flexor tendon injuries.

Facial anatomy

Eye

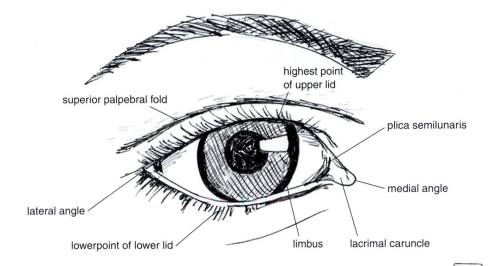

superior palpebral fold

highest point of upper lid

plica semilunaris

lateral angle

medial angle

lowerpoint of lower lid

limbus

lacrimal caruncle

The eyes lie at the junction of the upper and middle third of the face. The distance between the eyes is roughly equivalent to the width of one eye (actually slightly wider) or the root of the nose (actually slightly narrower). The curves of the upper and lower eyelids are different, the margin of the upper lid lies along the circumference of a smaller circle (2/3 of the radius of the lower lid). The highest point of the upper eyelid lies one third of the way from the medial canthus, whilst the lowest point of the lower lid lies one third of the way from the lateral canthus – at the medial and lateral corneal limbi approximately.

Proptosis – this is drooping of the eyelid when looking straight ahead. Normally the upper lid covers 2mm of the cornea.
Lid retraction – this is exposure of the sclera between the limbus and eyelid margin.

Lip

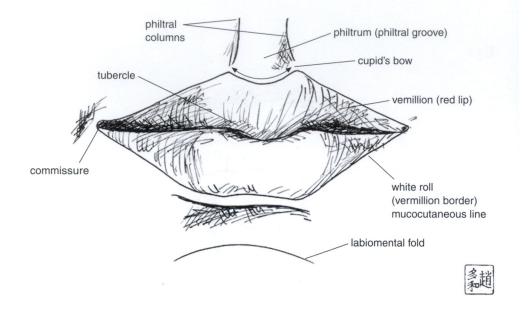

The vermillion is the red lip that owes its colour to the lack of a keratinized layer and the rich superficial vascular plexus; it has no sweat or sebaceous glands. The vermillion border represents the junction of skin and mucosa. The white roll is a subtle prominence adjacent to the vermillion border that reflects light. It is said that it is best to avoid cutting across the vermillion border where possible, and when it is unavoidable, then the incision should be perpendicular to the border. Precise alignment of the edge of the lip is vital as even a minor misalignment (1mm) is said to be noticeable. Another important landmark to preserve is the junction between the dry vermillion and wet vermillion.

Ear

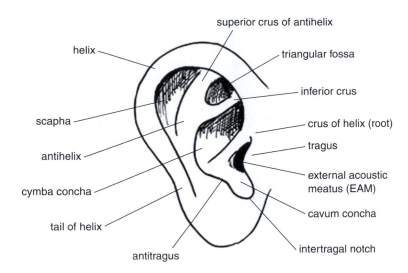

The axis of the ear is on average 20° which is roughly the incline of the dorsum of the nose – although the ear is usually more vertical. The superior attachment of the external ear lies just above the upper eyelid. The ear protrudes from the skull by about 20°.

Nose

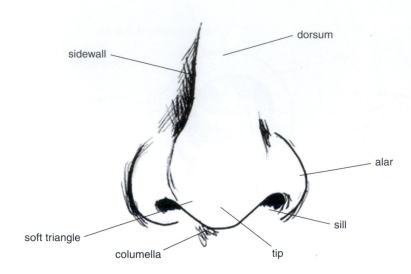

There are up to nine cosmetic subunits depending on whose description you read. It is said that if a defect is more than half the size of a subunit then cosmetic results may be better by replacing the entire subunit although not everyone follows this advice as it involves sacrificing 'good' skin.

The skin on the nose is not uniform in nature, it is thicker with many sebaceous glands on the tip and alar region, consequently skin grafts in this region may look more obvious. The underlying cartilages are very important in maintaining the shape of the nose.

Related topics of interest

Ear reconstruction.

Facial lacerations

Simple lacerations involving only skin

Pressure is the preferred method to control bleeding; 'blind' clamping is to be discouraged, as it may damage important structures.

- Irrigation of the wound with copious amounts of saline or water is a **vital** step and should be performed as soon as possible; its importance is often underestimated and omitted. High-pressure irrigation has been shown to be more effective in reducing bacterial numbers than low-pressure irrigation, but it may increase tissue damage; using a 20–50-ml syringe with a 16–19G cannula is sufficient in most cases. Antiseptics such as chlorhexidine are not necessary and may actually damage tissues.
- It is preferable to close wounds within 6h, but the good vascularity of facial soft tissue means that a slight delay is still acceptable (up to 24h).
- Regional block is preferred to local infiltration of local anaesthetic where possible. Avoid injecting directly into the wound. Debride skin sparingly, even 'questionably' looking, and trim grossly irregular or 'shelved' edges.
- Close in layers: deeper absorbable sutures should allow skin closure without tension. It is preferable to use 5-0 or 6-0 synthetic monofilament skin sutures to minimize tissue reaction, with particular attention to the precise apposition of the skin edges. The wound is waterproof after 48 hours. Sutures should be removed early (after 5 days for the face, after 3–4 days for the eyelids). Alternatives to sutures include tissue adhesives (cyanoacrylates such as Histacryl or Dermabond), which are particularly useful in children. It is important not to get the glue into the wound as it is cytotoxic. Steristrips are not as strong and come off easily when wet.
- Maximal wound strength (80%) is reached at 8 weeks.

Complex flaps are not indicated at this initial stage and any tissue loss that cannot be closed primarily is most appropriately treated with skin grafts. Abrasions are superficial wounds and will heal quickly, but need to be scrubbed thoroughly to avoid permanent tattooing that would be difficult to treat subsequently. It is important to establish the tetanus immunization status and treat appropriately.

Antibiotics are not needed unless the wound is contaminated or grossly infected; a lower threshold is sensible in those with immunosuppression, e.g. diabetics or those taking steroids. Prophylaxis has been shown to be effective (Cochrane review) at reducing infections in dog, cat and human bites. Augmentin is adequate in most cases.

- *Pasteurella canis, Pasteurella mulocida* in dog or cat bites
- *Eikenella corrodens, Streptococcus, Staphylococcus* and anaerobes in human bites, including puncture wounds on the knuckles from punching someone in the teeth.

Deeper lacerations
Knowledge of the underlying anatomy is invaluable for the plastic surgeon dealing with trauma:

- Muscle bellies can be apposed with a modified Kessler type stitch without excessive tension that would otherwise strangulate the tissues or 'cut through'. Muscle healing has been demonstrated in animal models.
- The parotid duct lies along the middle third of a line joining the tragus to the midpoint of the philtrum; it travels with the buccal branch of the facial nerve and the transverse facial artery. Lacerations of the parotid gland itself do not need to be sutured (salivary fistulae are rare and tend to close conservatively within a few days). In cases of suspected duct trauma, the duct is cannulated and then repaired with fine sutures over a stent that is either looped out of the mouth, taped to the face or cut short and secured intraorally. The stent is left in place for 5–7 days. If the duct cannot be repaired:
  —Stump ligation is recommended for proximal injuries. This will lead to temporary painful swelling with a small risk of infection; the gland subsequently atrophies after a couple of weeks. In general, the use of vein grafts to reconstruct the duct has been unsuccessful.
  —In distal transection, the duct stump can be diverted to the oral cavity, but it is a difficult and sometimes unrewarding procedure.

Facial nerve

The facial nerve exits the skull through the stylomastoid foramen and within 1.5 cm it splits into two main divisions, the temporofacial and cervicofacial, before forming the

Table 1   Effects of injury to various branches of the facial nerve.

Facial nerve branch	Surface landmarks	Effects of injury (main muscle affected)
Temporal	Along a line 0.5 cm below the tragus to 1.5 cm above the lateral eyebrow (Pitanguy) and becomes increasingly superficial	Brow ptosis, loss of forehead wrinkling (occipitofrontalis)
Zygomatic (most important)	Usually several branches that can be seen anterior to parotid and posterior to zygomaticus major	Lagophthalmos, exposed cornea (orbicularis oculi)
Buccal (multiple)	Parallel to and 1 cm below parotid duct	Lip weakness and lack of smile (zygomaticus, buccinator)
Marginal mandibular	Above a line 2 cm inferior to the mandible, deep to platysma and superficial to facial vein/artery	Unable to depress the corner of mouth (depressors anguli oris and labii inferioris)
Cervical	Deep to platysma	Clinically insignificant (platysma)

pes anserinus. There is significant crossover (70%) between the zygomatic and buccal branches and injuries to one are often well compensated for by the other. There is far less (15%) crossover with the other neighbouring branches. The location of the nerve branches and the effects of injuries are shown in Table 1.

Other nerves

The location of other nerves and the effects of injuries are shown in Table 2.

Table 2 Effects of injury to other nerves.

Nerve	Surface landmarks	Effects of injury
Supraorbital	Supraorbital notch lies 2.5 cm from the midline and above the midpupil (supratrochlear is 1 cm medial to supraorbital)	Numbness of forehead and upper eyelid (supratrochlear supplies the central forehead)
Infraorbital	Lies 1 cm below the orbital rim below the midpoint of the pupil	Numbness of side of nose, cheek and upper lip
Mental	Mandible below second premolar or corner of the mouth approximately. These three nerves lie on the same vertical line	Numbness of chin and lower lip
Great auricular	Located 6 cm below the external auditory meatus	Numbness of inferior half of the ear and angle of mandible

Further reading

Holger JS, Wandersee SC, Hale DB. Cosmetic outcomes of facial lacerations repaired with tissue adhesive, absorbable and non-absorbable sutures. *Am J Emerg Med* 2004; **22:**254–7.

Related topics of interest

- Local anaesthetics
- Suturing.

Facial reanimation

Facial expression is a function of both voluntary and involuntary action of the facial muscles. The motor supply comes from the seventh cranial nerve—the facial nerve.

Facial paralysis may be due to:

- **acquired palsy:**
  —Commonest cause is Bell's palsy and most cases tend to recover well.
  —Iatrogenic, e.g. following parotid or acoustic neuroma surgery.
  —Trauma.
- **congenital:**
  —Moebius syndrome: multiple cranial nerve palsies (especially abducens and facial nerves) with limb and pectoral anomalies. The cause is unknown.
  —Goldenhar: these patients have significant disability and deformity due to hemifacial microsomia and facial nerve palsy. It is often associated with dermoids.

When considering the restoration of facial nerve function:

- Duration of paralysis determines end-organ availability—after prolonged denervation, the muscle motor end plates will atrophy and then facial nerve restoration will be futile.
- The cause and level of palsy will generally determine the availability of proximal and distal nerve stumps for anastomosis.

Overall, the success of reanimation decreases with the age of the patient as well as with the duration of the paralysis.

Procedures can be divided into two categories:

- Dynamic—where movement, particularly a symmetrical smile, is the basic aim.
  —**nerve** restoration when the muscle still has potential function
  —**muscle** transfer, when the facial muscle is no longer functioning due to degeneration of motor end plates after prolonged denervation.
- Static—no additional movement is possible, but aims to produce a more acceptable resting face. Some procedures have a specific protective role.
  —Eye. Gold weight to upper lid, lower lid ectropion may need a lateral canthopexy, wedge resection or temporalis sling. A ptotic brow that obscures the lateral visual field can be lifted
  —Face. Lifts can be performed with fascia lata slings (corner of mouth, brow or forehead) that may have functional effects, e.g. brow (see above) and cheek (bringing the cheek against the teeth improves feeding and speech)
  —Botulinum toxin injection can reduce synkinesia, hypertonia and improve symmetry.

Dynamic facial reanimation

Nerve restoration
If both proximal and distal nerve stumps are available, e.g. after parotid surgery:

- Direct repair of nerve at the time of damage is likely to be very successful.

- Nerve grafting is best performed early (preferably within 6 months) and success rates approach 95%. If the facial nerve trunk is involved, synkinesia (mass muscular action) is likely to result due to the loss of individualized innervation of specific muscles.
  —The sural nerve (up to 35 cm available) or nerves of the cervical plexus such as the great auricular nerve (10 cm) are common donors for grafting. It is important to repair without tension as an additional 20% of shrinkage is expected and may compromise a tight repair. Repair by suturing the epineurium is preferable to fascicular repair.

If only the distal stump is available, then direct grafting is not possible, e.g. following intracranial/temporal surgery. Instead a 'donor' nerve is needed, either the contralateral facial nerve or others.

Cross-facial nerve grafting

- Cross-facial nerve grafting (CFNG) produces good results in early palsy in young patients. The repair is said to be 'physiological', producing good resting tone with symmetrical voluntary movements possible. Typically, a sural nerve graft is sutured to the contralateral facial nerve and the affected ipsilateral nerve stump. (The nerve graft is reversed to reduce 'axonal escape'.) The surgery may be done in one or two stages, with two-stage surgery being more common.
- In most cases, success is limited by the 'weak action' produced as only a quarter to a half of the axons will cross and there is less success with temporal and mandibular branches. The best results are achieved if the procedure is done very early (three months), however disadvantages include:
  —damaging the contralateral face and facial nerve and causing a donor defect
  —the nerve has to cross two suture lines
  —long overall denervation time for the muscle.

Nerve crossovers

Hypoglossal nerve crossover is popular after acoustic neuroma surgery. The glossopharyngeal (IX), accessory (XI), ansa hypoglossi and phrenic nerves can also be used.

- It involves only one suture line at the expense of a possibly significant donor defect: using the hypoglossal nerve will lead to moderate tongue atrophy in more than half of patients. There may be difficulty with speech articulation and handling of the food bolus during swallowing.
- There is a tendency to produce uncoordinated mass movements. The results are rather unpredictable but overall 80% have good results with improvements possible with intensive physiotherapy and training.

As such, crossovers are generally reserved for those patients not suitable for CFNG, e.g. for older patients in whom surgery is done after a lengthy delay (but with muscle still functional). It can be used as a temporary 'baby sitting' procedure to keep muscle 'toned' while awaiting CFNG. In these cases, usually only 30–40% of the nerve is used so that the donor deficit is less pronounced.

Muscle restoration

When facial palsy has been prolonged, restoring the nerve may be pointless as the end organ will no longer be functional due to end organ degeneration; at this point, functional muscle needs to be transferred. When this should happen depends in part on the age of the patient; it could happen at anytime from 1 to 3 years. An EMG is useful to assess the integrity of the end organ/muscle. If the facial nerve is potentially intact, the patient should be observed for at least a year before embarking on surgery. Even with the best results, there will still be a visible bulky mass that will get bulkier with contraction.

One cannot hope to reconstruct all the facial muscles; the basic aim is to at least reproduce the action of the zygomaticus major, which can produce an almost normal smile (albeit without the lateral and depressor function of the buccinator). The major drawback is that the size of the motor units in donor muscle is often ten times larger than the average facial muscle, making the resultant movement(s) much coarser.

Local donor muscle
- Temporalis can be turned over and slips transposed into the eye and mouth area. Additional grafts of fascia, e.g. fascia lata, may be needed due to the short muscle length. Training is required to obtain the best results.
- The masseter can be split into three slips to be inset around the oral commissure. The vector of contraction is more lateral than superior compared with the temporalis.
- Sternocleidomastoid is seldom used (bulky and unfavourable direction).

Free muscle
- Pectoralis minor is a popular choice for children. A multidirectional functional result is possible, but the muscle has a short variable pedicle, and the operation has a steep learning curve.
- Gracilis is unidirectional; it has a long consistent pedicle with a nerve supply from the anterior division of the obturator nerve. However, the muscle is rather thick and often needs debulking.
- Less common choices are latissimus dorsi, serratus anterior, rectus and platysma.
- Single stage procedure—the muscle is transferred and the motor nerve sutured to a facial nerve branch. One can use other recipient nerves such as the hypoglossal, but synkinesis would be more common with the latter.
  —only a single suture line with no donor defect from nerve graft
  —donor muscle suffers from prolonged denervation.
- Two stage procedure—this is preferred by many surgeons; the presence of nerve regeneraton at the stumps can be assessed histologically.
  —A reversed sural nerve is used as a CNFG and its end banked in the ipsilateral tragus.
  —After demonstrable regeneration (using an advancing Tinel's sign), free muscle is inserted with its nerve anastomosed to the CFNG stump.

Further reading

Ueda K, Harii K, Asato H, Yamada A. Neuromuscular free muscle transfer combined with cross-face nerve grafting for the treatment of facial paralysis in children. *Plast Reconstr Surg* 1998; **101:**1765–73.

Related topic of interest

- Botulinum toxin.

Flexor tendon injuries

Tendons are tough fibrous structures made of dense collagen bundles that connect muscles to bones. They are surrounded by endotenon and a loose layer of paratenon; there are few cells: tenocytes, fibroblasts and synovial cells. Flexor tendon injuries are common and have significant functional implications for the patient and must be treated properly.

- Flexor digitorum profundus (FDP) has four bellies, one for each finger. Tendons insert into the base of the distal phalanx.
- Flexor digitorum superficialis (FDS) has a common belly, although the index finger may have a separate belly. The tendons lie superficial to the FDP until the level of the proximal digital flexor crease where it decussates around the FDP (chiasm of Camper) and reforms to insert to the proximal half of the middle phalanx.

Digital flexor sheath

The flexor tendon sheath has two components:

- **Membranous**—a thin layer that covers the distal tendons in the hand. The closed synovial system forms bursae containing synovial fluid that has an important gliding/lubrication action and also contributes to the nutrition of the tendon.
- **Retinacular** or fibrous—there are condensations over the digital portion of the sheath called pulleys: five annular and three cruciate (see Table 1). They are important in preventing bow-stringing and in maintaining the mechanical advantage of the tendon.

The A2 and A4 pulleys are the most important and should be preserved if at all possible; they are broad and lie between joints, whereas the A1 and A3 are thinner and are found at joints.

Nutrition

There is much debate regarding the source of nutrition for the tendons of the hand.

- **Perfusion**—Blood supply to the tendons comes primarily from the vinculae (from the Latin 'vincio' to bind) that have segmental branches from the digital arteries. Vessels also enter the tendon at bony insertions. The vascularity is concentrated

Table 1 Position of the five annular pulleys.

Pulley	Position
A1	Over the metacarpophalangeal joint (MCPJ)
A2	Proximal phalanx
A3	Proximal interphalangeal joint (PIPJ)
A4	Middle phalanx
A5	Proximal to the distal interphalangeal joint (DIPJ)

mainly on the dorsum of the tendon and remains quite superficial in the endotenon septae. There is no overlap in flow between the territories of the vinculae and the supply to the tendons over the proximal phalanx, in particular, is poor. Presumably these areas are sustained by diffusion.

- Nutrients from synovial fluid can reach the tendon by **diffusion**; some propose that finger movements pump fluid into the narrow canaliculi that pass through the tendon. The FDP tendon is more dependent on diffusion than the FDS.

Current thinking is that diffusion is more important.

Zones

The level of flexor tendon injuries is classified into zones (Verdan, see Table 2). Note that these zones do not describe the level of the skin injury; the two do not necessarily match up and depend on the finger position at the time of injury.

Mechanism of tendon healing

Controversy exists regarding the mechanism(s) of healing:

- **Extrinsic**—It was initially thought that healing comes from fibroblasts producing peritendinous adhesions, and this theory was the basis for the immobilization regimes of the past.
- **Intrinsic**—Tendons bathed in synovial fluid were found to heal well; collagen is produced by tenocytes.

Similar sequence to fractures:

- **Haemostasis**—platelet deposition, vasoconstriction and fibrin
- **Inflammation**—there is an accumulation of inflammatory cells and cytokines that lasts up to a week

Table 2   Classification of flexor tendon injuries.

Zone	Position
Zone 1	Between FDS and FDP insertions—only the FDP tendon is found in zone 1
Zone 2	From FDS insertion to the A1 pulley. Dubbed 'no man's land' (by Bunnell): there are two tendons wound around each other within a tight tunnel. Repair is difficult and the risk of adhesions is increased. Around 50% of flexor tendon injuries are in zone 2
Zone 3	From the carpal tunnel (flexor retinaculum, FR) to the proximal A1 pulley. The lumbricals arise from the FDP tendons in this area
Zone 4	Carpal tunnel
Zone 5	From the muscle origin to the carpal tunnel

- **Proliferation**—(up to 1 month) fibroblast proliferation close to the cut tendon ends leads to deposition of disorganized collagen fibres with subsequent vascular ingrowth. There is also proliferation of epitenon cells that covers the injury to restore a smooth surface in a fashion analogous to a fracture callus.
- **Remodelling**—begins at about 6 weeks with a parallel reorientation of collagen fibres that increases the strength of repair. Hence, increased mobilization can start at this stage.

It was an important discovery that stressed tendons heal better with fewer adhesions and that greater excursion reduces extrinsic healing.

Management

History and examination are very important, as always. In terms of the history, patient hand dominance and occupation are important. Finger position during the injury determines the congruency between the level of the tendon injury and the skin injury.

Type of injury:

- open—lacerations or puncture, e.g. from teeth or glass
- closed, e.g. rugby jersey injury
- crush injuries have a wide zone of injury with possible associated injuries, increased risk of infection, repair failure/rupture and adhesions
- attrition, e.g. rheumatoid arthritis and fractures including Colles and scaphoid.

Examination

It is important to exclude other injured structures especially nerves and bones.

Diagnosis of tendon laceration
- In some cases, the lacerated tendon may be visible in the depths of the laceration. However, if the finger was flexed at the time, then the tendon injury may be significantly distal to the skin laceration.
- In closed injuries, there may be little to see apart from swelling and pain.

To aid diagnosis of a tendon injury, there are important clues from examining the resting position of the hand:

- **normal cascade of fingers**—composite flexion increases from index to little finger; if there is a flexor tendon injury then that finger will be more extended and disrupt the cascade
- passive manipulation of the wrist to examine the movement of the fingers extending and flexing due to **tenodesis** effect of antagonistic tendons
- **compression of forearm** flexors would normally increase the degree of finger flexion.

Partial tendon injuries are more difficult to diagnose and there is a risk of converting it to a complete injury during examination.

Specific examination of FDP and FDS

With the patient's hand palm up, other fingers fixed in extension by the examiner:

- FDS: patient asked to flex finger tip
- FDP: PIPJ and MCPJ of that finger fixed also, ask patient to flex the finger tip distal phalanx; 20% of patients have no FDS tendon to the little finger.

Remember also to examine for other injuries such as fractures and neurovascular damage.

Surgery

Note that not all patients should have their tendons repaired: this includes those who are uncooperative or have active infection. A failed primary repair is **worse** than no repair at all.

General principles

- Repairing within 6 h is the conventional teaching, but 12 h is also acceptable if antibiotics are used. Delayed surgery is possible; the patient may present late or ongoing infections may need to be treated first.
- Antibiotics and tetanus booster immunization as indicated.
- Repair under tourniquet control to improve visualization.
- Handle the tendons carefully; avoid handling uninjured areas and grasp only the end of tendon, taking care to avoid injuring the epitenon, otherwise adhesions may form.

Zone 2

Extended incisions are used to provide access for exposure while avoiding injury to neurovascular bundles.

- Brunner incision (volar zigzag)
- Bunnell (midlateral incision), either volar or lateral. Incisions on the ulnar side of the little finger or radial side of the index finger that are prone to contact should be avoided.

Tendon ends may not be immediately obvious.

- distal end may have retracted if the finger was flexed when injured
- proximal end may retract into the palm due to muscle tension. It can be retrieved by:
  —'milking' the tendon and flexing proximal joints
  —making an incision in the distal palmar crease (just proximal to A1), feeding a cannula down and pulling back after attaching tendon end to it.

There are many different repair techniques; they commonly combine:

- **Core suture**—usually a 3/0–4/0 monofilament, e.g. Prolene (some prefer to use braided sutures e.g. Ethibond), Kessler (parallel suture with locking) or Bunnell (criss-crossing) with at least four throws; 40% failures are due to knot slippage. Tendency to use increasing number of sutures to increase repair strength, but this also increases difficulty of surgery.

- **Epitendinous suture**—usually a 5/0–6/0 monofilament continuous suture; important that it only takes epitenon. It provides up to 20% of total repair strength. Outside zone 2, the epitendinous suture is less important.

The repaired tendon should have little or no bulk so that it can pass smoothly under pulleys. The surgeon should avoid damaging the A2 and A4 pulleys and should reconstruct them, if injured, with grafts from tendons or the extensor retinaculum (these grafts continue to secrete synovial fluid).

Zone 1

In the treatment of lacerations, if there is more than 1 cm of distal stump remaining, the tendon can be repaired conventionally, but this can be difficult due to a tight A4 pulley. If the stump is shorter, the tendon may need to be repaired onto the button on the fingernail. Some tendon injuries may be due to avulsion injuries; there may be a variable bone fragment involved that determines how far proximally the tendon retracts (see Table 3).

Other zones

These are simple repairs in comparison, but often multiple tendons are involved and there may be problems matching up tendon ends. In zone 3, it is important to take note to avoid suturing the lumbricals into the tendon repair.

The treatment of partial lacerations is described in Table 4.

Table 3   Classification of avulsion injuries.

Type of avulsion injury	Size of bone fragment	Position of proximal tendon
Type 1	No fragment	Palm—all blood supply has been severed; therefore, need early surgery (within a week) is advised. Scarring of sheath likely
Type 2	Small fragment	Tethered by vinculae, usually near the PIPJ. Surgery can be delayed up to 6 weeks because blood supply is intact
Type 3	Large fragment	Tethered by bone at A4 pulley. Can be repaired late

Table 4   Treatment of partial lacerations.

Partial laceration (%)	Recommended treatment
Up to 25%	Smooth down tendon flap that may otherwise catch in the sheath
From 35% to 50%	Running 6/0 epitendinous suture
More than 50%	Core suture and epitendinous suture

Postoperative care

Splintage
A dorsal block splint is used to keep the wrist 30° flexed and the MCPJ 90° flexed and IPJ neutral extension. The trend has been for the amount of flexion in the splint to be reduced.

Rehabilitation
The key factor in success is patient compliance with the various rehabilitation protocols available. Patients have to be aware that there need to be frequent regular visits to a physiotherapist and surgeon, and that unrestricted motion and normal use of the hand does not happen until 12 weeks after repair. Rupture of the repair is most likely in those who are mobilizing best. A repaired tendon actually becomes weaker immediately after the operation (5–21 days) and then gradually becomes stronger thereafter. Strength increases more rapidly when the tendon is stressed: stressed tendons also become stronger eventually and have fewer adhesions. For zones 1–3, early mobilization is recommended except for unreliable patients, children, poor quality tendons, e.g. crush injuries, and those with additional damage.

- **Duran**—controlled passive motion
- active
  - **Modified Kleinert.** Active extension within the limits of the splint and rubber band traction to provide passive flexion of fingers. Contractures can be a problem.
  - **Belfast.** Early active motion is currently favoured and provides good results, but with increased risk of rupture.

- better results outside zone 2 (85%) compared to 80% in zone 2
- poorer results if there are other injuries such as fracture or nerve transection.

Belfast regime (1989) (subject to many local modifications)

- Uses 4/0 monofilament Kessler with epitenon suture
- Dorsal block splint.

From day 2 to 6 weeks, every 2 h:
Passive flexion (to reduce contractures): apply gentle fingernail pressure to push fingers into palm ×2.
Active flexion (to limit fibrous attachment and increase strength of repair): active movement of IPJ joints, then mass movement of all fingers to gentle fist ×2; after each set, there should be active extension to touch splint with nails.
Six weeks: remove splint using active flexion exercises. Hand can be used but avoid heavy work
Eight weeks: slow increase in activity, fine work
Ten to 12 weeks: heavier work including driving
After 12 weeks: normal activities, only 60% strength at 16 weeks

---

A comparison of outcomes for the Belfast and Kleinert regimes is shown in Table 5.

Table 5 Outcomes for the Belfast and Kleinert regimes.

	Belfast regime	Kleinert regime
Risk of rupture	10%	5%
Good result	>80%	>70%
Contractures	Fewer	More
Patient acceptance	Compliance higher due to more supervision	Lower compliance

Complications

The commonest complication is adhesion, causing stiffness. If discovered early, then protocol modification is needed, otherwise flexion contractures will result. The risk of adhesions is increased by:

- trauma to tendon and sheath, e.g. crush injuries or 'heavy' intraoperative handling
- prolonged immobilization
- bleeding into sheath around repair
- sheath resection.

Other complications include:

- rupture, especially at postoperative days 7–10. If the diagnosis is uncertain, then MRI may be useful when range of movement cannot be used in assessment
- injury to neurovascular bundle
- infection
- reflex sympathetic dystrophy.

Further reading

Thien T, Becker J, Theis JC. Rehabilitation after surgery for flexor tendon injuries in the hand. *Cochrane Database Syst Rev* 2004; **4:**CD003979.

Related topic of interest

- Extensor tendon injuries.

Fractures of the mandible

The commonest causes of mandibular fractures are road traffic accidents and inter-personal trauma; consequently, patients show a male predominance (3×).

The condylar area is most frequently involved (29%); other commonly involved areas include the angle, the symphysis and the body of the mandible. Exact figures differ between sources, due in part to the different populations. The distribution of fractures is partly explained by pre-existing areas of weakness of the mandible (see Table 1).

The mandibule forms a ring-like system; therefore, in approximately 50% of cases there is more than one fracture (contre-coup fractures) (see Table 2): finding one fracture should prompt examination to specifically exclude others; there is an average of 1.5 fractures per mandible fracture.

'Favourable and unfavourable fractures'

An unfavourable fracture is a fracture in which the muscles tend to pull the fragments apart. In a favourable fracture, the fragments are pushed together by the muscle action.

- for those in a horizontal plane, the line runs downward and forwards
- for those in a vertical plane, the line runs from medial, forward and lateral.

With a trend toward open surgery, the significance of fracture favourability is reduced, but it remains a useful concept to rationalize the treatment in selected cases.

Table 1 Pre-existing weak areas of the mandible.

Weak area	Underlying reason
Condylar	Narrow thin bone of the neck
Angle	Third molar roots
Parasymphysis	Mental foramen and canine tooth root
Body	Bone is thin due to resorption and so this fracture is more common in the elderly. The body fractures nearer the angle in the edentulous

Table 2 Complementary mandible fractures.

Fracture	Complementary fracture
Condyle	Contralateral angle
Angle	Contralateral body
Parasymphysis	Contralateral condyle
Symphysis	Bilateral condyles

Assessment

Initial assessment should always follow ATLS guidelines, i.e. ABC:

- Airway. Obstruction may be caused by the backward displacement of fracture fragments or from excessive bleeding; such fractures may need to be distracted and fixed.
- Breathing. There may be coexisting chest injuries such as tension pneumothorax or flail chest.
- Circulation. There may be profuse bleeding from fractures. Treatment may involve packing, reduction or arterial ligation if necessary.

Specific assessment

Diagnosis of the fracture is part of the secondary survey. Severe concomitant injuries should be excluded before the facial fractures.

- Any deformity may be masked by swelling and bruising; there may be crepitus. Gently but thoroughly palpate the bony margins for focal tenderness or step deformities.
- Check maxillary and facial stability.
- Assess the degree of mouth opening. Trismus (less than 35 mm opening) may be due to spasm or direct trauma to the muscles.
- Wear facets are useful clues to check for problems with occlusion; many patients do not have 'normal' pre-trauma bite (angle classification).
    —Class I (74%)—the mesobuccal cusp (anterolateral of the four cusps) of the upper first molar fits into the buccal groove (the groove between anterior and posterior cusps) of the lower first molar
    —Class II (24%)—mandibular retrognathia
    —Class III (1%)—mandibular prognathia.
- Intraoral examination for haemotomas (almost always seen in fractures) swelling and lacerations: a significant proportion of mandibular fractures involve the teeth and overlying mucosa and are classed as 'open'. These are prone to infection, and prophylactic antibiotic treatment is recommended. Penicillins or cephalosporins are the drugs of choice.
- Check for trigeminal distribution numbness or paraesthesia, especially of the chin and lower lip.
- Associated injuries are not uncommon (45%):
    —There is a 3% chance of concomitant spinal fracture in patients with major injuries of the face.
    —10% have eye injuries.
    —Skull base fracture may be indicated by CSF rhinorrhoea or epistaxis.

Imaging

- The best single plain radiograph is an orthopantomogram (OPG or Panorex). Older films had problems with reduced symphyseal detail, but these have largely been resolved. Subcondylar/condylar and the ramus are not as well visualized as the rest of the mandible.
- A 'mandibular series' of plain radiographs is a reasonable alternative if OPG is not available. (OPG requires special equipment and a stable patient).

—Caldwell—PA view with 15° tilt to remove the shadow of the petrous temporal bones from the orbit

—Oblique view showing ramus and adjacent body

—Towne or reverse Towne—AP with 30° tilt that provides a submental view demonstrating the subcondylar region by protecting it below the mastoid.

- Computed tomograms (CT) are of limited routine use, but may be indicated for surgical planning or for confirming diagnosis if clinical suspicion remains high despite equivocal X-rays, especially for suspected condylar fractures. Note that a CT entails 20 times the radiation dose of a plain X-ray.
- Others:

  —A chest radiograph is advisable if missing teeth are unaccounted for.

  —Dental occlusal views.

Treatment

- Nurse head up to reduce swelling
- Antiseptic mouthwash e.g. chlorexidine
- oral antibiotics if the fracture is open.

Conservative treatment may be appropriate in selected cases:

- children, especially with greenstick fractures
- 'favourable' undisplaced fractures with normal occlusion and minimal trismus
- subcondylar fractures, especially if undisplaced.

Otherwise the general trend is towards operative repair where possible.

Intermaxillary fixation (IMF)

This term is explained by the fact that the mandible used to be called the inferior maxilla. Wires and arch bars are used to fix the mandible to the maxilla after occlusion is restored.

- IMF is a non-rigid form of fixation. It has been the traditional treatment for mandibular fractures and gives reasonable results. It needs to be in place for 4–8 weeks if used alone. It is not effective for severe bony displacement and non-union is more common than with mini-plates.
- It is a significant undertaking for the patient: oral hygiene needs to be meticulous. There are potential airway problems and the patient may find it difficult to maintain weight through oral feeding.
- It is generally not recommended for those with poor compliance, those suffering from epilepsy or other seizures or psychiatric illness, for those who are pregnant, children or for those with multiple injuries (especially head injury).

Open reduction and internal fixation (ORIF) is generally regarded as the treatment of choice as it allows open visualization and precise reduction—IMF is recommended to fix the occlusion first. Unicortical fixation is preferable to bicortical fixation to reduce root damage, particularly in children. If the fracture line lies anterior to the mental foramen then two plates are required, otherwise one plate is sufficient. Rigid fixation avoids prolonged immobilization that may cause temporomandibular joint (TMJ stiffness) and allows early rehabilitation but may lead to stress shielding and is technically more demanding.

Table 3 Types of fixation and mechanisms used.

Types of fixation	Mechanism
Rigid	Lag screws, compression plate
Semi-rigid	Miniplates
Non-rigid	IMF, splintage

The types of fixation and the associated mechanisms are shown in Table 3.

External fixation was commonly used during the Second World War, but is seldom used now except for selected situations such as compound or comminuted fractures in the edentulous elderly patient.

The timing of surgery depends on several factors:

- Operating within 48 h reduces the rate of infection, but there is little demonstrable difference in clinical results between this and operating within a week. It is often not possible to arrange the necessary investigations and the operating time before significant swelling occurs. Consequently, surgery will need to be delayed until the swelling reduces, which may take several days. Two weeks is probably the practical upper limit for primary surgery, but the young heal at a faster rate.
- Late secondary surgery requires osteotomy and may be difficult due to soft tissue contraction.

Complications of fixation
- Infection (6%) is the most common complication. It presents a major problem and may lead to non-union
- Non-union (3%), pseudoarthrosis
- Nerve injury (2–8%), particularly of the inferior alveolar nerve.

Condylar fractures

Treatment of condylar fractures presents a particular problem. Surgery access is often difficult with a risk to the facial nerve and TMS. Conservative treatment with soft diet for 2 weeks is suitable for most patients. ORIF is indicated in particular situations: e.g. if the patient is unable to maintain occlusion with conservative treatment, if there is severe angulation or lateral displacement of more than 30° with severe malocclusion, in patients with bilateral fractures and shortening (only one side needs to be fixed), or when there are foreign bodies in the temporomandibular joint. Intra-articular fractures may lead to ankylosis, probably due to haemorrhage leading to fibrosis.

Further reading

Vural E. Treatment of adult subcondylar mandibular fractures: closed vs open vs endoscopic approach. *Arch Otolaryngol Head Neck Surg* 2004; **130:**1228–30.

Related topic of interest

- Facial lacerations.

Gynaecomastia

This is the enlargement of the male breast; it can be a source of embarrassment and may be painful. Sometimes it may indicate severe underlying disease such as tumours: testicular, lung, pituitary, renal/adrenal and breast.

Figures regarding the frequency and incidence of the condition are variable, reflecting the lack of standard definitions of the condition. The age of onset is important in determining the most likely cause of the enlargement.

Pubertal (40%)

A small amount of breast hypertrophy accompanying the adolescent growth spurt is common, and may be regarded as 'physiological', possibly being due to an imbalance in the sex hormones. It is seen in up to two-thirds of 14 year olds. The problem is typically asymmetric and sometimes tender. It is usually self-limiting and most cases resolve within 6–18 months and does not warrant extensive investigation. The exception is where there is a marked increase (>4cm)—there is a secondary cause in 20% of these cases and endocrine evaluation is indicated. A similar type of enlargement occurs in neonates and elderly men; neonatal gynaecomastia is due to excessive maternal and/or placental oestrogens and usually disappears within weeks. Those with simple gynaecomastia do not have an increased risk of breast cancer.

Prepubertal

Gynaecomastia at this age is of more concern and warrants evaluation by a paediatric endocrinologist. Investigation may reveal:

- Reduced testosterone—**Klinefelters** patients have a 50× increased risk of breast cancer; typically such boys are tall, with reduced secondary hair and small genitalia; hyperthyroidism and congenital adrenal hyperplasia are other possibile causes.
- Raised oestrogen—true hermaphroditism, testicular tumours.

Adult

Enlargement in adults is usually due to excess fat with or without glandular hypertrophy. It often occurs in **healthy men**.

- Drugs may be responsible in some cases: alcohol, steroids, cimetidine, marijuana, tricylics, spironolactone, digoxin, diazepam, etc.
- Abnormal liver function/mild cirrhosis may be found, with abnormal steroid hormone handling.
- In hyperthyroidism, there is reduced circulating testosterone due to increased plasma binding proteins.

Routine endocrine screening of adult patients with gynaecomastia tends to be neither cost-effective nor particularly revealing.

Management

The history should concentrate on the following points:

- Time of onset
- Drug history
- Other symptoms suggesting systemic disease or malignancy, including weight loss.

Examination should aim to ascertain the presence/absence of:

- Thyroid disease
- Liver disease
- Genital problems.

Breast cancer is suggested by a hard eccentric lump, especially if there is skin dimpling.

Treatment

Nonsurgical treatment
- Correct reversible causes
- Depending on the cause, medication may help:
  —anti-oestrogens—clomiphene (variable response)
  —dihydrotestosterone—cannot be broken down to oestrogens
  —tamoxifen—good for pain, but less effect on size; more effective for enlargement of recent onset. Side effects include nausea.
  —Danazol—reduces pain and size due to its anti-gonadotrophin effects.

Surgery
- Liposuction alone is not very good because tissue is often fibrous/glandular; it may be a useful supplement to surgery in certain cases. Ultrasound-assisted liposuction may be more effective.
- Postoperative seromas and haematomas are relatively common; extensive surgery warrants placement of drains, preferably through the incision site to avoid an extra scar, and a pressure dressing.
- Endoscopic excision through an axillary incision is a recent development that may be suitable for selected cases.

Classification
The treatment is related to the grade or severity of the problem in terms of degree of enlargement and skin excess (see Table 1). Many different incisions have been described and each have their own advantages and disadvantages. All tissue that has been removed should be sent for histological examination.

Table 1 Grades of gynaecomastia and associated treatment.

Grade	Description	Treatment
I	Small enlargement as a localized button, no skin excess	Easy to treat with excisional surgery: button removed through 'classical' semicircular inferior circumareolar incision (Webster). Liposuction may be useful
IIA	Moderate diffuse enlargement, no skin excess	Removing diffuse enlargement is more difficult and prone to causing 'dishing', a sunken effect. This may be reduced by combining tapering the edge of excision (through an extended Webster incision) along with liposuction. There may also be waviness of the skin postoperatively due to fat necrosis
IIB	Moderate enlargement, excess of skin	Doughnut mastopexy
III	Marked enlagement with excess skin	Larger degrees of enlargement require a large incision line that extends beyond the areola • breast reduction type incision (Letterman technique) • horizontal ellipse +/− free nipple graft

Further reading

Wiesman IM, Lehman JA Jr, Parker MG et al. Gynaecomastia: an outcome analysis. *Ann Plast Surg* 2004; **53:**97–101.

Related topics of interest

• Breast reduction
• Liposuction.

Hair removal

Excessive hair is a common cosmetic problem that can affect healthy individuals; the 'normal' amount of hair for an individual is related in part to their ethnicity, and cultural factors determine its acceptability. Excessive hair may sometimes be due to hormonal disturbance, most commonly hyperandrogenism from exogenous or endogenous causes (sources, ovarian or pituitary).

- Congenital adrenal hyperplasia
- Polycystic ovary syndrome
- Hirsuitism—this is excessive growth of hair in females in a male pattern. Most cases show a genetic predisposition and the problem is usually oversensitivity to androgen rather than over-secretion
- Hypertrichosis—this is excessive growth of hair in a non-androgen distribution that is above normal for the age, sex and race of the patient. It can be congenital or acquired, such as drug-induced (cyclosporin, phenytoin and minoxidil).

Even cases labelled 'idiopathic' may have a subtle hormonal overactivity or oversensitivity.

Assessment of the patient requires a full history and examination; those with a suspected hormonal problem should be referred to the appropriate specialists.

Hair cycle
It is important to appreciate that hairs grow and rest in cycles:

- Anagen—growth phase. The duration of this phase determines the length of the hair. Different areas of the body have different lengths of cycle and not all hairs in one area will be in the same phase
- Catagen—transition
- Telogen—resting.

Methods of hair removal

Shaving. This is simple but needs to be repeated every day or so; there is also a risk of cuts and irritation. Contrary to popular myth, hairs do not actually increase in number after shaving.

Depilation. Thioglycolates are used to disrupt the disulphide bridges in keratin and the hair breaks above the skin surface. Irritation or allergies may occur.

Epilation. This is removal of the entire shaft by various means. The long-term effects on hair growth are unclear, but hairs may become finer with repeated damage to the matrix.

- Waxing is one of the most effective methods and effects can last for several weeks. It is more effective when performed by experienced practitioners. Honey is used in a similar way.
- Plucking by hand with tweezers or with machines is similar in principle. 'Threading' is practiced by some cultures in China and the Middle East.

- Electrolysis is the insertion of fine needles into the follicle to damage it. There is a theoretical risk of causing infection.
  —DC current—'galvanic' electrolysis causes chemical damage by generating sodium hydroxide.
  —AC current—'thermolysis' is thermal damage due to vibrational energy. Most modern equipment uses this mode alone or in combination with galvanic mode in 'blend' machines—caustic damage is seen to be greater when combined with heat.

Temporary reduction of hair

Eflornithine hydrochloride (Vaniqa) is applied as a cream, and by inhibiting ornithine decarboxylase, it reduces hair growth after several weeks of use. It works in about half of patients and as it does not actually remove hair, it has to be combined with the hair removal techniques described above. Hair will return when the treatment is stopped.

Laser hair removal

Lasers have proved to be very useful in hair removal. The pluripotential cells responsible for hair growth are in the bulge/bulb region that lies some 4 mm below the skin surface. These cells are destroyed by heat conducted from the melanin in the follicle (the chromophore). Only hair follicles in the anagen stage are vulnerable to laser energy, and since hair follicles are at different stages of the hair cycle, laser treatment must be repeated to catch more hairs in the anagen stage.

There are many laser systems available for hair removal:

- long-pulse ruby (694 nm)
- long-pulse alexandrite (755 nm)
- long-pulse diode laser (810 nm)
- long-pulse Nd-YAG (1064 nm)
- intense pulsed light (IPL 500–1200 nm).

However, long-term studies on the effectiveness of laser hair removal are lacking. The hair colour needs to be darker than the skin colour for lasers to be most effective. A frequent concern in the past used to be causing hyperpigmentation in darker skins, but modern machines are safe enough to be used on most skin types (though caution is still required in darker skin types). Longer wavelengths are used for better skin penetration and offer better protection for epidermal melanin; Nd-YAG is better for darker skins, but not as good for lighter coloured hairs. Cooling systems are used in many current laser systems to protect the skin further.

- Cooling gels
- Contact cooling—the pressure of contact also helps to displace haemoglobin from the treatment site
- Cryogen spray is delivered in a controlled manner before each pulse.

Pre-treatment preparation
- Patch testing is important to determine the optimal fluences to be used; there should be hyperaemia, mild swelling and some pain, otherwise the energy is going to be inadequate for hair removal.
- Topical anaesthesia is usually needed. Popular choices are EMLA (lignocaine and prilocaine), Ametop (amethocaine) and newer creams include 4% and 5% lignocaine.
- Sun-tanning and waxing/plucking just before laser treatment should be avoided.

Post-treatment
- A mild sunburn-like appearance with mild oedema may last for 3–7 days.
- Ejection of hairs occurs for 2 weeks after treatment.

The commonest complication is hyperpigmentation that may last for several months. Significant scarring is rare.

Patient satisfaction is usually good, but **promises of 100% effect or zero regrowth are false**.

- Individual responses cannot be predicted. Many have a good result but some will have poor results.
- Usually 2–3 treatments are needed to catch the majority of hairs in the anagen phase, but some regrowth is always possible—on average 80% clearance is expected.
- **Painless treatment** (without topical anaesthesia) is ineffective at producing permanent hair removal. Permanent damage to the follicles only comes at energies that cause pain, otherwise the follicles are simply pushed into the resting phase (telogen) for a period of dormancy before returning. Sublethal laser energy may alternatively cause regression of the terminal hair vellus hair (miniaturization).

Further reading

Lepselter J, Elman M. Biological and clinical aspects in laser hair removal. *J Dermatolog Treat* 2004; **15:**72–83.

Related topic of interest

- Lasers: principles.

Hypoplastic facial conditions

There is a range of conditions associated with facial hypoplasia (abnormally small face). Reconstruction is complex and involves many operations.

Treacher–Collins syndrome

Treacher–Collins syndrome (TCS or mandibulofacial dysostosis) is associated with bilateral first and second arch abnormalities. The 'Treacle' gene on chromosome 5 is implicated and inheritance of the condition is autosomal dominant with variable penetrance; clinical expression is highly variable. Prenatal diagnosis by chorionic villus sampling or amniocentesis is available. Children have distinctive features with a convex shaped facial profile and look 'fish-like'. The IQ is normal; any developmental delay present may be related in part to hearing loss.

- Eye and ear abnormalities:
  —coloboma, loss of medial lower lashes, anti-mongoloid slant, strabismus and hypertelorism
  —microtia, cryptotia, narrow ear canals, middle ear abnormalities; 95% have hearing loss (usually conductive).
- Hooked/beaked narrow nose and long side burns. There is an association with cleft lip/palate; those who do not have a cleft may have a high arched palate. Some have abnormally shaped heads without true craniasynostosis.
- Hypoplastic midface/maxilla and mandible including the temporomandibular joint (TMJ) is the central feature; mandibular hypoplasia in combination with choanal atresia can cause severe airway compromise at birth.
  —The airway may be managed simply by nursing prone, but may require a tracheostomy or formal mandible surgery such as augmentation, and sputum. Sleep apnoea is a common problem.

Hemifacial microsomia

There are a number of alternative terms including craniofacial microsomia, otomandibular dysostosis or first or second branchial arch syndrome. Most cases are sporadic with a variable degree of clinical expression and may be related to stapedial artery thrombosis; a few familial cases have demonstrated various modes of inheritance. It resembles TCS but can be distinguished from it because it is usually asymmetrical (though it is bilateral in 10%). Less than 5% of cases have the characteristic features of Goldenhar's syndrome, with vertebral anomalies (e.g. fused or hemivertebrae) particularly in the neck region, benign growths around the eye (epibulbar dermoids). The classical facial features of hemifacial microsomia can be summarized by the acronym OMENS (see Table 1).

Distraction osteogenesis relies on the formation of bone in the gap between the gradually distracted bone ends of a corticotomy. A fixator is used to gradually distract the bone ends at a rate of approximately 1 mm per day.

Table 1 Facial features of hemifacial microsomia.

	Problem	Treatment
Orbit	Anophthalmia, ophthalmoplegia, epibulbar dermoids	Advancement
Mandible	Hypoplasia leading to tilted occlusion and chin deviation	Reconstruction with bone or costochondral grafts or distraction techniques
Ear	Microtia, sensorineural hearing loss	Staged reconstruction, hearing aids
Nerve	Facial nerve palsy	May need two-stage operation with sural nerve grafting and muscle transfer
Soft tissue	Deficiency of 5th and 7th nerve muscles, macrostomia	Flaps for soft tissue augmentation. Cheek may need bone augmentation. Commissuroplasty

Hemifacial atrophy of Romberg

There seems to be no strong evidence of genetic inheritance with most cases being sporadic; presentation is very diverse. There is progressive wasting of one side of the face and forehead that in the majority begins before the patient reaches their 20s and lasts for 7 years on average before burning out, leaving hypoplasia and atrophy. The disease primarily affects the subcutaneous tissue and fat.

- En coup de sabre—sharp indentation across face and extending to hairline, with localized hair loss affecting the scalp, eyebrow and eyelash
- Skin may show atrophic changes, hyperpigmentation or vitiligo
- Neurology: epilepsy, migraine and trigeminal neuralgia.

Patients show a slight female predominance; the right and left sides of the face are affected with equal frequency. There is evidence that some form of autoimmunity causes hyperactivity of brain stem sympathetic centres leading to the atrophy. It resembles a localized form of scleroderma and there are antinuclear antibodies present in some cases.

No treatment has been shown to stop the progression of the disease. Surgery is postponed until the condition has burnt itself out and has been stable for at least 6 months (usually longer). There have been anecdotal reports of flaps atrophying if transposed while the disease is still active. As a general rule, bony abnormalities are corrected first before the soft tissue is filled in various ways including free flaps. It is advisable to overcorrect to take account of subsequent atrophy with any debulking delayed for at least 6 months.

Further reading

Wang RR, Andres CJ. Hemifacial microsomia and treatment options for auricular replacement: a review of the literature. *J Prosthetic Dent* 1999; **82:**197–204.

Related topic of interest

- Craniosynostosis.

Hypospadias

In this condition, which occurs in one in every 300 live Caucasian births, an abnormally proximal urethral meatus is found in the ventral aspect of the penis or less commonly, the scrotum. There has been an increasing incidence over recent years, which may be explained in part, but not entirely, by increased awareness and surveillance. Other features include:

- dorsal hooded prepuce
- chordee is a fibrous band that may cause a curvature either at rest or only during erection. The deformity is more pronounced in the more proximal forms of hypospadias. Chordee can be assessed intraoperatively by the artificial erection test (with a tourniquet applied and sterile saline injected into the corpora)
- paraurethral sinus, urethral valves and flattened glans.

Half of the patients also have inguinal hernias and one-fifth may have undescended testes.

Apart from the cosmetic issues, there may be certain functional problems:

- unable to micturate standing up
- reduced fertility:
  —deposition of semen in the female reproductive tract may be hindered
  —severe degrees of chordee make penetration painful or difficult.

There is a 10% risk in first-degree relatives. Both babies of an identical twin pair are not always affected, thus implicating environmental factors in its causation. Androgen receptor deficiency or an increase in exogenous oestrogens may be important. Babies born from in vitro fertilization are at five times higher risk of having hypospadias, and this may be related to maternal progesterone levels.

Hypospadias is generally classified according to the position of the meatus (after correction of any chordee). There are a number of classification schemes, with some variation:

- distal or proximal
  —85% are distal (glandular, coronal, subcoronal, distal penile shaft)
  —15% are proximal (midshaft, proximal penile shaft, penoscrotal, scrotal and perineal).
- distal, middle or proximal
  —distal (50%) glandular, coronal, subcoronal
  —middle (20%) distal penile, midshaft or proximal penile
  —proximal (30%) glandular, coronal, subcoronal.

The subcoronal position is commonest. Chordee is more common with proximal femur.

Assessment

Important aspects of the physical examination include:

- assessing penis size

- verifying testicular descent
- observing urine flow (if possible).

The presence of hernia should be specifically excluded, and if present, further investigation of the urinary tract is warranted.

Surgery

Surgery aims to provide the patient with a normal-looking penis with normal sexual function and a normally positioned urethral meatus with a normal urinary stream. It is important not to have the boy circumcised before surgery.

Timing
- Previously, surgery was delayed until the patient was 3 years old or older: the larger penis size theoretically allowed easier surgery and the patient had better comprehension and cooperation.
- Current practice aims to perform surgery at 8–12 months for one-stage surgery or slightly later for two-stage surgery. Fitness for surgery is the primary limiting factor.
- Operating at 2–3 years of age is generally avoided due to a perceived increase in psychological adjustment problems.

Chordee correlation involves dealing with either a fibrous subcutaneous band or a problem with the corporea. Those with the severest variants may need a multistaged procedure. The urethra is repaired where possible using the urethral plate but with insufficient tissue, there are many techniques available to reconstruct the urethra with other tissue.

Techniques
There are many techniques available—they generally fall into the following categories:

- single-stage techniques
- two-stage techniques.

Single-stage techniques
The urethra is reconstructed with vascularized tissue as onlay (incomplete tube that is completed by the urethral plate) or inlay tube grafts (complete tube). The tissue can be transposed:

- as a reflected flap: onlay (Mathieu, 'flip-flap') and inlay (Mustarde)
- as an islanded preputial flap: onlay or inlay (Duckett).

Two-stage techniques
Bracka (modified Cloutier)

- During the first stage, performed at around 1 year of age, the glans is split longitudinally and the defect covered with an inner preputial skin graft.
- The second stage is performed 6 months later, when the graft is tubed over a catheter in two layers.

There are obvious disadvantages of having to undergo two operations, including the extra cost and the additional general anaesthesia. However, there is some controversy regarding the actual amount of psychological trauma suffered as it seems that it is the final appearance of the genitalia that has a greater impact than the number of operations.

Two-stage operations provide good cosmesis with a slit-like meatus that is less likely to stricture by avoiding a circumferential anastomosis. There is a quoted fistula rate of 3%. The operation is technically simple and reliable; it is versatile and suitable for revision surgery.

Advancement techniques are suited for selected patients, with distal defects. These were often ignored because of a lesser extent of function problems.

- MAGPI (Duckett) **M**eatal **A**dvancement and **G**lanulo**P**lasty **I**ncorporated is suitable for very distal meatuses. A longitudinal incision is made distal to the abnormal meatus and closed transversely to provide some advancement.
- BEAM (**B**ulbar **E**longation and **A**nastomotic **M**eatoplasty). The meatus is advanced by dissecting free a length of penile urethra. Up to 5 cm in adults and 2.5 cm in children can be advanced with this technique.

Complications

The complications commonly encountered during treatment of hypospadias are shown in Table 1.

Table 1 Complications encountered in treating hypospadias.

Early	Late
• Erections, particularly in young adults, can disrupt the surgery and are suppressed by commencing cyproterone acetate 10 days before surgery • Wound infection and dehiscence are less common with the routine use of prophylactic antibiotics • Bladder spasm from the catheter	• Stenosis—15% usually require further surgery • Fistula rate—15% overall, risks are increased in revision surgery. Most appear early (within a week) and rarely close spontaneously • Recurrent urinary tract infections, especially if hairy skin was used to graft the urethra

Further reading

Manzoni G, Bracka A, Palminteri E, Marroco G. Hypospadias surgery: when, what and by whom? *BJU Int* 2004; **94:**1188–95.

Informed consent

In the absence of evidence of consent, the doctor leaves himself open to claims of negligence (breach of duty) or assault and battery. More importantly, it is the duty of every doctor to empower their patients to allow them to make informed decisions.

Forms of consent

- Express—this means that agreement for the particular procedure or investigation has been sought and given verbally or in written form. This is recommended for procedures with significant risk and also if research is being conducted.
- Implied—the patient cooperates without specifically agreeing to the procedure. It is important to note that compliance is meaningless by itself and does not equate to consent if the patient does not understand the procedure or if they are not aware that they can refuse.

Capacity to consent

It should be assumed that everyone is able to consent unless it can be shown otherwise; in England, Wales and Northern Ireland, no one can make decisions on behalf of a competent adult.

- **Mental incapacity**—in England, relatives cannot can give or refuse consent on behalf of a mentally incapacitated adult. The doctor determines what would be in the 'best interests' of the patient (and fits in with the opinion of the majority of his or her peers): the family may advise and support the decision. In the USA and many other countries, a proxy decision maker can be appointed, being either the patient's legal representative or a family member (spouse > adult child > parent > adult sibling > adult grandchildren) but only if the decision is in the best interests of the patient.
- **Child (under 18)**—in general, a parent can authorize treatment even when a competent child may refuse (one exception is Scotland, where a legal process would be needed to overrule the competent child's refusal). When parents refuse a procedure in the child's best interest, then application to the court is needed to proceed. There is some variation in local laws.
- **Emergencies**—in an emergency, doctors can provide care without consent, but this is limited to saving the patient's life or to preventing significant irreversible deterioration. The doctor must respect any previous wishes, e.g. living wills, made when the patient was competent.

Consent forms are almost universal, and while they are advisable legally, they only represent evidence of the process—that some discussion has taken place—rather than the process itself. Discussions should be recorded in as much detail as possible in the patient's notes.

An important part of the doctor–patient relationship is **trust**. To facilitate this, the doctor must respect a patient's autonomy, remembering that patients have the legal right to make decisions about their health care and to determine what treatment to have or whether or not to undergo the medical intervention suggested. To allow patients to make informed decisions, doctors must provide sufficient information in a clear manner. Continual open dialogue helps establish what the patient wants and needs to know, then an agreed framework can be achieved.

It is the duty of a doctor to ensure that the essential components of the process of informed consent are provided:

- An explanation of the patient's condition is provided, along with the likely prognosis if it is treated or left untreated.
- Any uncertainties in the diagnosis should be made clear with an explanation of the value of further investigations.
- The purpose of the proposed treatment or investigation is stated, with an explanation of the procedure including the probability of success and the risks of failure. Side effects should be discussed: include the *common even if not serious and the serious even if uncommon*. Alternative treatment should be included in the discussion.
- Declaration of the experimental nature of a procedure, if applicable.
- It is important to remind patients that they can seek a second opinion and can change their minds at any time.

The doctor providing treatment is responsible for ensuring that consent has been correctly obtained. An experienced doctor, preferably the doctor performing the procedure, should obtain consent from the patient, but the task may be delegated to someone who is trained and has sufficient knowledge/familiarity with the procedure. The possibility of problems requiring additional treatment coming to light during a procedure when the patient is unconscious or otherwise incapacitated should be discussed; any objections or limits to this must be established.

How much information is actually given depends on the patient, and it is the doctor's duty to determine the patient's priorities, which will be affected by their beliefs and culture. Sufficient time should be given for the patient to digest information, particularly after bad news. The patient should be asked specifically if they understand; a relative or close friend may be useful to support the patient and reinforce the information subsequently. Obtaining consent is not an isolated event; because of the dynamic nature of disease, it is important to review the discussion, particularly just before a procedure.

Patients' questions should be answered with honesty; the doctor should not deliberately withhold information. Particular care and attention is needed when obtaining patient consent for screening tests as there may be wide-ranging consequences; a positive result or even undergoing the screening itself can have significant implications for the patient. It is important to make the patient aware that false-negative or false-positive results can occur.

Refusal

Competent adults are entitled to refuse consent even when it may lead to their death or serious/permanent injury.

Further reading

General Medical Council. Seeking patients' consent: the ethical considerations. London: GMC, 1998.

Keloids and hypertrophic scarring

Dermal injury triggers a cascade that results in the deposition of a vascular collagen matrix that, as it accumulates, becomes a red, raised **scar**. As the matrix matures and remodels, the scar will become flatter and paler after 9 months (takes longer in children). However, sometimes healing does not follow the usual pattern and excessively lumpy raised scars occur. These scars fall into two main categories:

- Hypertrophic scars, which seem to follow a similar, but protracted, course to normal scars along with a tendency to involute.
- Keloids (from 'cheloide' after the Greek 'chele' for a crab claw to describe its lateral extension) appear after a delay and have a tendency to increase in size and spread laterally.

Apart from the unsightliness, there may be additional symptoms of itching and discomfort. In large complex lesions, there can be a risk of recurrent infection.

These types of problem scarring follow a variety of injuries, and anecdotally there is:

1. predilection for certain sites, i.e. ears, shoulders, pre-sternal and upper band, crossing skin tension lines. Conversely, some areas seem to have inherently low risk: palms/soles, eyelids and genitals
2. relationship with wound infection
3. relationship with wound tension during closure.

These associations may be stronger in hypertrophic scars compared with keloids.

Differences from normal scars

Both hypertrophic scarring and keloids show histological differences from normal scars: they are more vascular and have thicker epidermal layers; in addition, the matrix contains more type III collagen and has collagen nodules that are not found in mature scars.

Differences between keloids and hypertrophic scars

There are differences between keloids and hypertrophic scars in their clinical characteristics and response to treatment. Much has been written, but it is important to bear in mind that:

- very few published studies have a sound methodology; lack of randomization and inadequate follow-up are the commonest shortcomings
- many studies do not properly distinguish between keloids and hypertrophic scars.

History is important in determining the stage in the evolution of the scar. Keloids and hypertrophic scars can look very similar—histological differences are said to exist but can be so subtle that distinction is not always possible. See Table 1 for a comparison of keloids and hypertrophic scars.

Table 1 Comparison of hypertrophic scars and keloids.

	Hypertrophic scar	Keloid
Onset	Usually occur early, within weeks/months	May be delayed up to several years
History	Tends to regress with time	Tends to progress with time
Extent	Stays within the boundaries of the original wound	Extends beyond the boundaries of the original wound
Microscopy	Wavy loose bundles of collagen. More fibroblasts • collagen synthesis is 3× normal scar • collagenase activity is 4× normal scar	Disorganized sparse bundles of large irregular collagen fibres with reduced cross-linking. Even more disorganized and more ground substance than hypertrophic scars • collagen synthesis is 20× normal scar • collagenase activity is 14× normal scar

Keloids

The overall risk of having a keloid scar is estimated at 5–15%, but accurate and reliable figures are not available. Keloids are more common in darker-skinned people; a keloid diathesis may run in families with evidence of loci on chromosomes 2 and 7. Overall there is little information on why keloids occur.

- reduced apoptosis and increased proliferation of fibroblasts
- role of TGF beta and IGF-1 in the formation of keloids.

While 'spontaneous' keloids have been described, the majority actually follow a known but trivial problem such as a pimple/acne. Truly 'spontaneous' keloid formation is probably an extremely rare phenomenon.

Treatment

There is a range of treatments used for both keloids and hypertrophic scarring; the underlying reasons for their action has not been fully elucidated. Proper comparison is made difficult because:

- most studies do not distinguish between keloids and hypertrophic scarring
- lack of standardized treatment regimes.

Because hypertrophic scarring tends to regress spontaneously, it can be difficult to judge when treatment is actually successful as opposed to natural regression of the lesion.

- **Pressure**—may work through local tissue hypoxia/ischaemia. Tailored garments are designed to deliver around 24 mmHg of pressure and need to be worn for prolonged periods. Older scars respond less well. It is probably more useful in hypertrophic scars than keloids.

- **Silicone gel**—may work by occlusion and hydration of the scar surface. If used for 24 h a day for 3 months, the response rate is approximately 65–88%. There is little evidence for its use in the prevention of problem scarring.
- **Steroids**—the reported response rate varies widely from 30–100%. The optimal concentration is not clear; triamcinolone (kenacort) is available in concentrations of 10 mg/ml and 40 mg/ml. Some practitioners use lignocaine to improve comfort; intralesional injection is very painful. Local side effects include dermal thinning/atrophy, telangectasia and pigment changes. Systemic effects such as endocrine disturbance and osteoporosis are rare. The value of topical steroids is unclear.
- **Excision** or ablation by surgery, cryotherapy or laser have all been used but are generally considered to have similarly high rates of recurrence (more than 50%), although figures are sketchy. Re-excision of a scar may be worth considering if there were specific problems such as infection. Surgery is probably best combined with other modalities such as steroids, pressure or radiotherapy to reduce the risk of recurrence.
- **Lasers**
  —Ablating with CO_2 or argon lasers has a recurrence rate similar to surgery.
  —Nd-YAG lasers are reported to have variable effectiveness.
  —Vascular lasers such as the pulsed-dye laser (PDL) may be effective for itching and redness, particularly in hypertrophic scars. It is said to act by reducing the microvascular perfusion that leads to breaking of the collagen disulphide bond with subsequent reformation in a more orderly fashion.
- **Radiotherapy** inhibits fibroblast proliferation. Early (24–48 h) postoperative administration of a single dose (10–14 Gy) reduces the rate of recurrence compared to surgery alone, although there is no role for radiotherapy alone. Malignant complications (thyroid malignancies) have been reported only rarely but must be a consideration in the young.

Less commonly used treatments include:

- immune response—interferons (gamma for hypertrophic scarring, alpha 2b for keloids) and the immunomodulator, imiquimod
- chemotherapeutic agents—5FU, bleomycin, mitomycin C
- controlled lathyrism—penicillamine, colchicines, BAPN
- miscellaneous—antihistamines, Retin A.

There is very little objective information on the effectiveness of these less-common treatments.

Further reading

Ragoowansi R, Cornes PG, Moss AL, Glees JD. Treatment of keloid by surgical excision and immediate postoperative single-fraction radiotherapy. *Plast Reconstr Surg* 2003; **111**:1853–9.

Related topic of interest

- Lasers: principles.

Lasers: principles

Lasers are rapidly developing into invaluable therapeutic tools. However, there is a rather common misconception among patients and doctors alike: that lasers are some sort of modern technological wonder that can deal with all manner of skin problems without any side effects.

Problems can subsequently arise when patient expectations are unrealistic, particularly in terms of efficacy, safety and the side effect profile. It is vitally important to understand the physics and principles of lasers; this permits improved decision-making, better patient counselling, and the safe and effective use of the technology.

L.A.S.E.R. (Light Amplification by Stimulated Emission of Radiation)

When an excited atom spontaneously returns to the resting state, it will emit a photon of a certain wavelength. If this photon hits another atom in the resting state it will raise it to an excited state; however, if this photon hits an atom in an already excited state then two photons are released.

What a laser system provides is:

1. An external energy source that increases the proportion of excited atoms held in the laser medium.
2. An arrangement of mirrors (a fully reflecting mirror at one end and a partially reflecting mirror at the other) that allows the light emitted to be reflected back and forth.

This allows light energy to be **amplified**.

A laser will deliver energy in the form of **collimated**, **coherent** and **monochromatic** light (see Table 1). When such light impinges on body tissue, the light will be transmitted, scattered, reflected or absorbed to differing degrees, depending on the relationship between the wavelength of the light and the absorption characteristics of the tissue.

When laser light is absorbed, it is usually converted to heat (photothermal interaction), leading to a range of temperature-dependent effects. In other situations, depending on the intensity and duration of energy transfer, the light energy can lead to photomechanical or photochemical interactions (see Figure 1).

Basic laser technology constitutes a very precise and controllable source of intense heat. Its suitability for clinical use involves matching these properties to the problem, and this is where experience is crucial.

Table 1 Basic terms used to describe the properties of laser lights.

Collimated	Single direction
Coherent	Single phase
Monochromatic	Single wavelength

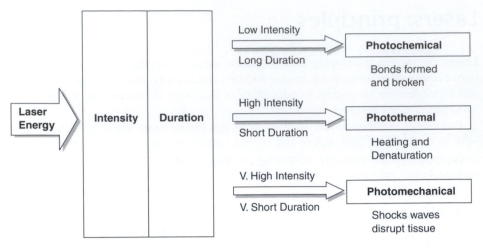

Figure 1 Tissue effects of laser light.

Photothermal effects: the CO_2 laser

The carbon dioxide (CO_2) laser was one of the first lasers to be used for medical purposes and remains a 'workhorse' used in many areas of surgery as a result of its versatility. Its wavelength of 10600 nm preferentially targets water in the tissues, where heating leads to destruction ranging from denaturation and necrosis to vaporization, depending on the **fluence** (=energy density in J/cm²) delivered.

A defocused CO_2 laser beam can be used to ablate or vaporize lesions; however, when focused into a narrow beam, it cuts like a scalpel with excellent haemostasis (except for larger-calibre or high-flow vessels). On the other hand, compared to 'cold steel', equipment costs are high, the process is relatively slow and initial healing may be slower.

Applications of lasers in plastic surgery

If the inherent properties of a particular laser can be matched to the clinical problem, then lasers can be used with good effect in a variety of conditions with relatively few complications and side effects, and as such represent significant advances over conventional methods (see Table 2).

Table 2 Clinical conditions treated by laser.

Condition	Typical laser used
Skin resurfacing	CO_2, erbium-YAG
Pigmented lesions	Q-switched ruby, alexandrite, Nd-YAG
Tattoos	Q-switched ruby, alexandrite, Nd-YAG
Hair removal	Long-pulse ruby, alexandrite, diode
Vascular lesions	Pulse dye laser (PDL)

CO_2 lasers are **precise, but non-specific**—they cannot be used to destroy pigmented or vascular lesions without causing damage to surrounding and overlying normal tissue, leading to a significant risk of scarring. Problems can potentially occur because it is impossible to limit exactly the amount of damage and where the damage occurs. An element of collateral damage is unavoidable, but in excessive amounts, it will increase the risk of scarring and other complications.

Selectivity of lasers

Several conceptual advances have improved the understanding of lasers and made their clinical application much more logical.

> *Selective thermiolysis* is the targeting of a specific tissue component to be heated and destroyed without damage to neighbouring tissues. Central to this is the concept of the *thermal relaxation time* (TRT), which is the time for the target to cool to 50% of the maximum temperature rise without conducting heat to the surrounding tissue.
>
> Thus, if the rate of heating is greater than the rate of cooling, then the target is heated, leading to its destruction before significant conduction to surrounding tissues. On the other hand, if the rate of heating is less than the rate of cooling, then both target and surrounding tissue is heated, and the effect is less specific.

Chromophores (coloured molecules) in the skin will absorb light of a particular wavelength. Heating can be effectively *restricted* to the target chromophore if laser light of a suitable wavelength and appropriate pulse duration is chosen. Something close to a 'magic bullet' is achieved: only the target is damaged with no collateral damage.

However, this holy grail of perfect selectivity is not possible because the other chromophores will absorb some of the energy. For example, when targeting haemoglobin with a PDL, some of the 585-nm light will also be absorbed by melanin (leading to dyspigmentation) and by water (leading to non-selective skin damage—pain and erythema). Thus, unwanted effects cannot be totally eliminated, but the correct choice of laser parameters may minimize these.

> **Chromophores** (coloured molecules)
>
> - Melanin in skin and hair
> - Haemoglobin
> - Exogenous pigment (tattoos)
> - (Water).

Further reading

Rosenberg GJ, Gregory RO. Lasers in aesthetic surgery. *Clin Plast Surg* 1996; **23**:29–48.

Related topics of interest

- Hair removal
- Tattoo removal
- Vascular anomalies.

Leg ulcers

An ulcer is a break in the skin and may have many different causes. In developed countries, venous disease (more than 75%) is the most frequent cause; however, biopsy should be performed in chronic cases to exclude malignancy.

Venous ulcers

Venous ulcers take up a large part of the health budget. These are classically found in the 'gaiter' area (a gaiter is a protective piece of cloth or leather covering the area from the instep to the ankle), particularly in the medial malleolus. Venous hypertension is commonly caused by valve dysfunction, which itself is usually caused by previous thrombophlebitis. Prolonged tissue hypertension leads to extravasation of proinflammatory protein-rich exudates into the tissues resulting in scarring (lipodermatosclerosis) and hyperpigmentation.

Proper assessment is vital to guide management appropriately.

History and examination:

- Ulcer characteristics, especially the edge and base
- Exclude malignancy: remember to examine the regional lymph nodes
- Surrounding skin and the circulation of the limb
- Sensation (diabetic neuropathy is suggested by glove and stocking distribution).

Investigations

- It is important to biopsy long-standing lesions.
- Wound swabs may be useful, but colonization is common and antibiotics are generally unnecessary unless there is evidence of clinical infection: pus, increased pain, fever and spreading cellulitis.
- Ankle brachial index (ABI). Readings of <0.8 suggest arterial disease, whereas an ABI of <0.5 should prompt referral to vascular surgeons.
- X-rays may be indicated to exclude osteomyelitis.

For those with suspected **venous disease**, duplex scanning is the non-invasive investigation of choice, although superficial reflux is often the only finding. For those with suspected **arterial disease**, angiography is recommended.

Management

Treatment depends on the cause: venous ulcers are generally treated non-surgically with elevation, compression and dressings. Most will heal if the venous hypertension is controlled. However, there is a tendency for these to recur (40%).

- Ulcers can be washed with tap water. Debride necrotic material adequately.
- There is a whole range of dressing materials available: simple non-adherent dressings may be used (there is little evidence that others offer significant advantages). Hydrocolloid/foam dressings may be useful to reduce pain.

Table 1 Appearance and treatment of different kinds of ulcers.

Cause	Appearance	Surrounding skin	Typical distribution	Treatment
Venous There is often a history of DVT	Shallow ulcer with flat or slightly swollen borders. Fibrin/slough over a raw weeping base. Painless unless infected	Itchy, swollen, eczema, pigmentation, lipodermatosclerosis, atrophie blanche. Aching and swelling at the end of the day that is improved by elevation. Capillary refill less than 3 s	Gaiter area (between malleolus and lower calf) especially malleolus	**Compression.** Most will heal if venous hypertension-controlled Pentoxifylline has not been shown to provide significant benefit in randomized trials
Arterial Claudication is often a prominent symptom	Dry, deep punched-out (well circumscribed). Base is pale and may be covered with necrotic eschar and sparse granulation tissue. Pain worse with elevation and at night	Cold, shiny and atrophic (less hair). Pulse is weak. Capillary refill more than 4–5 s	Sides and toes, and dorsum of foot	**Revascularization** is required in most; amputation may be required Cilostazol, type II PDE inhibitor, improves claudication but not yet a recommended treatment for ulcers
Neuropathic Diabetes, alcoholism, leprosy, tabes dorsalis and spina bifida	Painless. Look similar to arterial ulcers but variable in depth	Surrounded by callus, may have sinuses. Paraesthesia or numbness with repeated trauma causes ulceration	Commonly, but not exclusively, at pressure points, e.g. Plantar surface beneath metatarsal heads, heels	In the absence of ischaemia, 90% heal without surgery Control infection Becaplermin gel with recombinant PDGF is an adjunct for diabetic ulcers

- Avoid topical antibiotics (often become sensitizers); systemic antibiotics are used for spreading cellulitis or preoperatively if grafts are used.
- Graduated, multilayer, high-compression bandaging provides a sustained 40 mmHg of compression at the ankle to reduce capillary transudate. It is kept intact for up to a week (if ABI >0.8). Seventy per cent will heal within 6 months; graduated stockings can be used to reduce the risk of recurrence (but need to be replaced every 6 months).
- Vacuum wound closure may be useful in some cases.

There are regional differences in practice: in the UK there is a preference for four-layer bandaging, in the US the Unna boot is popular and in Europe short-stretch bandaging is often used. There is no evidence that there is much difference among these.

If an ulcer fails to heal after 12 weeks of standard treatment, then this should prompt further assessment to rule out other causes, such as: vasculitis, infection, autoimmune disease, sickle cell or a tumour.

Surgery

Surgery is generally reserved for cases where conservative treatment has failed or if pain is a prominent symptom and is poorly controlled. Simple excision with grafts or flaps without addressing the underlying problem(s) is prone to recurrence; surgery such as subfascial ligation of perforators for reflux disease, for example, may be indicated.

Table 1 shows the appearance, distribution and recommended treatments for the different kinds of ulcers.

Further reading

Collum N, Nelson EA, Fletcher W, Sheldon TA. Compression for venous leg ulcers. *Cochrane Database Syst Rev* 2001; **2:**CD000265.

Related topic of interest

- Vacuum wound closure.

Liposuction

Liposuction is one of the commonest cosmetic procedures performed (also known as 'liposculpture'). It can be used to reduce focal deposits of adipose tissue that are unresponsive to diet or exercise, but also:

- for lipomas, particularly larger ones
- for Madelung's disease (multiple symmetrical lipomatosis) with deposits of unencapsulated adipose tissue, generally said to be commonest in male alcoholics
- as an adjunct in abdominoplasty, gynaecomastia and lymphoedema.

Subcutaneous fat is divided into superficial and deep compartments:

- The superficial layer has a densely packed fibrous stroma with horizontally and vertically arranged septae.
- The deeper layer is less compact with a sparse septum that is less well organized. This layer is primarily responsible for the shape of the body contour and liposuction is generally directed toward this deeper layer. Neurovascular bundles are protected by the stroma and are relatively safe from damage.

Fat cells do not increase in number in the adult, but remaining cells can hypertrophy; adipocyte numbers are fixed after adolescence unless there is morbid obesity (body mass index >39).

Types of liposuction

Liposuction techniques can be classified according to the amount of fluid infiltrated as well as the type of aspirator used.

Types of suction
- A vacuum (of approximately 1 atmosphere) sucks fat into the openings of a cannula, avulsing the fat; the procedure is repeated in two planes (cross-tunnelling). A syringe or pump can be used to create the vacuum; using a syringe is less traumatic, causes less blood loss and allows faster healing, but a pump is more efficient.
- Ultrasound-assisted liposuction (Zocchi) uses a suction catheter with 20-kHz mechanical vibration at the tip that induces fragmentation of fat that is then aspirated by the low-level vacuum. The tip needs to be kept moving constantly due to the danger of causing burns or perforations. The technique decreases the effort required and allows more fat removal, but it takes longer. Its advantages over conventional aspiration may be more apparent when there is also significant fibrous tissue such as on the buttocks or in gynaecomastia in particular.

Fluid infiltration
Prior to the development of tumescent/superwet techniques, liposuction required a general anaesthetic and the end point was often excessive bleeding (the blood loss could be as high as 40% of the aspirate), and patients were often asked to donate some of their own blood a month before.

Tumescent/superwet liposuction has made the procedure much safer:

- Only 1–3% of aspirate is blood due to the vasoconstrictor effect.
- There is no need for a general anaesthetic. Longer-lasting anaesthesia up to 24 h postoperatively is possible. Even when 35 mg/kg of lignocaine is used, maximum *plasma* levels at 11–15 h are only half of toxic levels at most. The absorption of lignocaine is slower due to the vasoconstriction.

Adding fluid also allows a smoother mechanical action. Superwet techniques involve smaller volumes than the tumescent techniques and thus have relatively fewer problems with fluid overload, but the lower dose of adrenaline (epinephrine) means slightly greater blood loss. While clearly superior to dry and wet liposuction, the advantages of tumescent over superwet liposuction (and vice versa) are unclear, but then modern liposuction tends to be a combination of the two.

The main problem is fluid balance due to the large volumes infiltrated. The procedure is contraindicated in patients taking medication that is also metabolized by cytochrome p450 such as cimetidine, erythromycin, beta blockers, etc., as there is an interaction that increases the potential toxicity of lignocaine. Hyaluronidase hastens the onset of action but may make absorption less predictable. Steroids are used by some but have been shown to have no effect on pain and may actually increase the rate of infection.

Table 1 gives the details of infiltrate and blood loss for different types of liposuction.

Table 1   Techniques for liposuction with and without fluid infiltration.

Technique	Infiltrate	Blood loss
Dry	None	May have significant blood loss, up to 40% of aspirate, hence no longer practiced
Wet (1980s Illouz)	Infiltration of 200–400 ml saline per average area liposuctioned	Blood loss around 20% of aspirate, reduced further to 15% by addition of adrenaline (Hettler 1983)
Superwet (1986 Fodor)	One millimetre of infiltrate per millimetre of aspirate, using saline, adrenaline and lignocaine	Reduces blood to 2–4 ml per litre of aspirate
Tumescent (Klein 1987)	Infiltrate to skin turgor (2–3 ml/ml aspirate) • 1 litre of saline/lactated ringers • 1 ml of 1:1000 adrenaline (giving 1 in 10^6) • 50 ml of 1% lignocaine • Bicarbonate (variable). Many variations, but few studies to determine which is best	Less blood loss, 1–2 ml per litre of aspirate

Complications of liposuction

- In very large series, there is a quoted 0.1–0.5% major complication rate. There have been isolated reports of deaths from pulmonary embolism, fat embolism and necrotizing fasciitis. The risks are increased with liposuction of extensive areas, or if combined with other procedures. It is better to stage liposuction procedures: avoid aspirating more than 1.5 litres at one sitting, otherwise the pathophysiology will resemble a large burn, and avoid combining with other surgical procedures.
- Fluid overload.
- Less serious problems include:
  —contour irregularity
  —damage to neurovascular structures causing haemorrhage, bruising, paraesthesiae and skin trauma.

Further reading

Commons GW, Halperin B, Chang CC. Large-volume liposuction: a review of 631 consecutive cases over 12 years. *Plast Reconstr Surg* 2001; **108:**1753–63.

Related topics of interest

- Abdominoplasty
- Gynaecomastia
- Lymphoedema.

Local anaesthetics

Cocaine is an alkaloid extracted from cocoa leaves and was the first local anaesthetic (LA) used. It is an effective anaesthetic agent with additional vasoconstriction that is useful in certain situations, but significant side effects, such as euphoria and addiction, limit its medical use essentially to operative preparation for treatment of the nose and throat. Procaine (Novocain) was a synthetic analogue (1905) that did not have the same problems with addiction but had other significant problems of its own—it had a weak action, it took a long time to work and was short acting. Furthermore, a high frequency of allergic reactions (up to 33%) means that it is no longer in common use.

Current commonly used anaesthetics include:

- **Lignocaine** (lidocaine) was developed in Sweden in the 1940s and is a good anaesthetic, although it has a vasodilatatory effect that increases the rate of systemic clearance. Therefore it is often combined with adrenaline (epinephrine) to prolong its effect.
  - —**Vasoconstrictors—adrenaline:** By reducing local blood flow, systemic absorption of the LA is reduced and thus its action is prolonged. This reduces the dose required and consequently the risk of toxicity is also reduced. The time for onset of action is 5–7 min depending on the concentration. A concentration of 0.8–1 in 1 000 000 is sufficient, and no benefit is seen in increasing the concentration beyond 0.8–1 in 100 000. A concentration of 1 in 200 000 is perfectly adequate for most clinical situations.
  - —Adrenaline can be safely used in local flaps (studies have not shown increased failure rates except in delayed flaps). The usual recommendations are to avoid use in fingers, toes, penis, nose and ears—although use is fairly common in the last two sites in particular.
  - —There is a risk of arrhythmias. Its use is contraindicated in phaeochromocytoma, severe hypertension, hyperthyroidism and severe peripheral vascular disease.
  - —The use of adrenaline has been shown to increase infection rates in contaminated wounds in vitro; reduced blood flow decreases leukocyte numbers and hypoxia reduces their function, especially the killing function. The in vivo effect is unclear.
- **Bupivicaine** is longer acting than lignocaine, but a slow onset of action limits its wider use. It has higher risk of toxicity; a direct effect on Purkinje fibres can promote re-entry and negative inotropy.
- **Prilocaine** has a duration of action similar to lignocaine but it is less toxic. It is generally considered to be one of the safest LAs, and is therefore recommended for intravenous regional anaesthesia, i.e. Bier's block. It has less of a vasodilatatory effect and can be used without vasoconstrictors, also making it theoretically safer to use in patients taking antihypertensives or on thyroid hormone replacement. It is also a constituent of EMLA. However, it can cause methaemoglobinaemia in susceptible individuals; this is a rare complication that can cause cyanosis, tachypnoea/dyspnoea and can lead to death.
- **Amethocaine** is a potentially toxic ester that is generally only used topically in ophthalmic drops and as Ametop for cannulation sites in children. It has some advantages over EMLA—it is cheaper, quicker acting (30 min) and longer lasting, It

causes vasodilatation and so facilitates cannulation. In addition, it can be used in younger children (even in premature babies) than EMLA can due to a lower risk of methaemoglobinaemia.

Action of local anaesthetics

LAs produce reversible blockade of voltage-gated sodium channels by binding to a site on the inside of the neuron axon. It affects pain 'C' fibres first as these are thin and unmyelinated.

LAs are generally weak bases and there is an equilibrium between the non-ionized form and the ionized charged forms. While it is the uncharged form that can cross lipid membranes, it is the charged form that is active and binds to the target. Lignocaine is about 25% diffusible at body pH; in abscesses or in areas of inflammation, where the pH is lower (typically 5–6), the amount of the diffusible form is much reduced and efficacy is poorer. Lipid solubility influences potency and the speed of onset.

Types of local anaesthetics

Examples of LAs and their metabolism are described in Table 1.

It is important to avoid toxicity from overdosing the patient; this requires knowledge of the maximal doses, which are related to body weight, but also requires adjustments in the presence of liver and renal disease. Toxicity may be potentiated in pregnancy or at the extremes of age.

- **Early** signs of toxicity include light-headedness, tinnitus, circumoral numbness and a metallic taste—these early signs may be missed if the patient is sedated/anaesthetized. Cardiac effects such as negative inotropy and arrhythmias may be particularly resistant to treatment.
- **Intermediate** signs include anxiety and tremors.
- **Late** signs include seizures and coma.

The commonest cause of toxicity is inadvertent intravascular injection.

Table 1 Metabolism and examples of local anaesthetics.

Types	Examples	Metabolism
Esters	Amethocaine, benzocaine, cocaine	Metabolized by plasma pseudocholinesterases. Related to PABA (para-aminobenzoic acid) and can cause allergy in one-third of patients. Most cases of allergy are minor with temporary itch or rash
Amides (two 'I's in the name)	Lignocaine, prilocaine	Metabolized by liver. Excretion in urine

Table 2 Clinical characteristics of lignocaine and leupivicaine.

Local anaesthetic	Onset	Maximum dose (adrenaline)	Duration (+adrenaline)
Lignocaine	Rapid (4 min)	3.5–4.5 mg/kg (7 mg/kg)	1–2 h (2–4 h)
Bupivicaine	2–10 min	2.5 mg/kg (3 mg/kg)	4 h (8 h)

The time until onset, the maximum dose and the duration of action of two commonly used LAs are given in Table 2.

- **1% = 10 mg/ml**, therefore one can give $4 \times 50 = 200$ mg or 20 ml of 1% plain lignocaine in a 50-kg patient.
- Lignocaine will still work at 0.25% but onset will be delayed.
- Adrenaline will still work at concentrations of 1 in 1 000 000 but will take longer; in practical terms, no more than 1 in 200 000 is needed in most situations. The addition of adrenaline increases the maximal doses of lignocaine that can be used but has less of an effect on bupivicaine. As a general guideline, do not inject more than 20 ml of 1 in 200 000 adrenaline in 10 min.

Tumescent anaesthesia is a technique that uses large volumes of solution with dilute lignocaine and adrenaline and allows up to 35 mg/kg to be infused into the subcutaneous tissue without ill effects; it seems that the vasoconstriction significantly delays the absorption of the LA to safe levels.

Potential problems using LAs:

- **The area injected does not become numb**—for blocks, this may be an error of technique, but in rare cases may also represent anomalous anatomy. True resistance to local anaesthetics is rare, but has been reported on occasion.
- **Severe pain**—a shooting pain may occur if the nerve has been hit by the needle. Withdraw the needle—do not continue with the injection in that location. There may be prolonged numbness lasting weeks/months but usually no permanent damage results.
- **Prolonged pain/numbness/paraesthesia**—this may be due to direct injury to nerves, which is a particular risk when infiltrating after partial/previous block. In addition, there is individual variation in the susceptibility to the drug. If the drug has been inadvertently injected under the periosteum, forming a reservoir, the effects may be prolonged.
- **Ischaemia** with pain and blanching may be due to inadvertent intra-arterial injection of adrenaline. The half-life of adrenaline is 2 min and usually no permanent damage results. The risk may be reduced by aspirating prior to injection—for this reason, 'dental syringes' are considered to be not as 'safe' as using standard syringes although they are convenient and have finer needles.
- **Tachycardia**—injection of vasoconstrictor into the circulation may quicken the pulse or cause arrhythmias, but this usually passes within a minute or two.

Reducing the pain of injection
- Warm the anaesthetic, e.g. warm to near body temperature by holding it, rather than using it straight from the refrigerator.

- Use a needle of the smallest calibre possible and minimize the number of times you need to enter the skin. Try to inject sequentially so that you inject through partially anaesthetized skin.
- Inject slowly.
- Avoid inflamed areas. Efficacy is reduced and there is an increased risk of infection.
- Part of the burning sensation is due to the low pH (4–5) caused by the preservatives—0.1 ml of 1.26% bicarbonate added to each ml of local anaesthetic; this will also speed up the onset of action. Due to the need to add bicarbonate manually, it is relatively inconvenient and is susceptible to errors.
- Mixing LAs may improve profiles, e.g. fast acting yet long duration; toxicities are not additive but the overall value is not proven.

Topical anaesthetics

EMLA (**e**utectic **m**ixture of **l**ocal **a**naesthetics—2.5% prilocaine and 2.5% lignocaine) is often used to anaesthetize the skin of cannulation sites, especially in children, but unfortunately it does not reduce apprehension. (Eutectic means that it is a mixture with a melting point lower than either constituent alone.) The speed of action varies by site depending on blood flow: on the face, some effect is evident after 15 min, but in other areas it may take up to 60 min. Roughly 1 mm depth is anaesthetized per 30 min up to a maximum of 5 mm at 120 min (90 min with 30 min wait) and the anaesthesia lasts 3–4 h. It has an essentially unwanted vasoconstrictor effect that potentially makes cannulation more difficult; this effect lasts for 30–90 min and is followed by vasodilatation after 180 min. Due to the prilocaine, there is a risk of methaemoglobinaemia in sensitive patients and its use is therefore not recommended in the very young. It needs to be applied generously and covered with Tegaderm—some cream should be visible at the end of the administration period otherwise it means that insufficient quantities were used.

Alternatives include:

- Ametop (4% amethocaine)
- ELA-Max 4 (4% lignocaine)
- ELA-Max 5 (5% lignocaine).

Further reading

Seigel RJ, Vistner LM, Iverson RE et al. Effective haemostasis with less epinephrine: an experimental and clinical study. *Plast Reconstr Surg* 1973; **51**:129–33.

Related topics of interest

- Facial lacerations
- Liposuction
- Suturing.

Lymphoedema

Lymphoedema is the abnormal collection of protein-rich fluid in the interstitium causing swelling. The cause is a reduced efficiency of lymph clearance due to an underlying lymphatic problem that may be congenital (primary) or acquired (secondary). The disease is limited to tissues superficial to deep fascia.

> The lymphatic system returns proteins and fluid that have accumulated in the interstitial space to the venous system; 100% of the total body albumin is recirculated every 48 h. The process is essentially passive.

The presence of protein-rich fluid in the interstitium triggers a vicious cycle making the disease progressive.

- The disruption of oncotic pressure promotes further accumulation of protein-rich fluid that is prone to infection. Phagocytic efficiency is reduced.
- The protein promotes inflammation and fibroblast activation leading to fibrosis, which causes hypoxia and further fibrosis.
- When the condition becomes chronic, the skin changes are typical: dryness, hyperkeratosis, lymphangiomas and cracks/fissures.
- **Lymphangiosarcoma**—Malignant transformation is said to become a significant risk (10%) after 10 years of disease. It occurs in 0.5% of those with lymphoedema after mastectomy (Stewart–Treves syndrome). The prognosis is poor and may require amputation.

Differential diagnosis

- Oedema—fluid excess is commonly due to renal or cardiac causes. Low protein states (nephritic syndrome, malnutrition or cirrhosis) generally cause a puffy oedema.
  - —Early lymphoedema may pit, but subsequent fibrosis abolishes this phenomenon.
  - —Elevation improves simple oedema quicker than it does lymphoedema.
  - —There are fewer skin changes such as thickening and ulceration in oedema.
- Obesity (lipoedema/lipodystrophy).
- Venous oedema is due to deep venous disease.

Lymphoedema is generally classified by cause, but this has little practical significance in terms of treatment.

Primary
No precipitating cause is found—it is a diagnosis by exclusion. There are subsets defined by the age of onset. Patients are often female (2:1).

- **Congenita** (20%) involves the lower limb most frequently, and one-third of cases are bilateral. Milroy's disease is a familial subset that may be due to lymphatic aplasia. It is inherited in an X-linked dominant manner with onset at puberty and may be associated with Turner's syndrome.

- **Praecox** (70–80%)—onset usually at puberty but can occur from age 14–35; lymphatics are hypoplastic in most cases.
- **Tarda** (10%) is a less common variant with later onset, typically after 35 years of age. Vessels are hyperplastic—tortuous and abnormal.

Secondary

Secondary lymphoedema is much more common:

- **Malignancy**—either primary lymphatic neoplasm or secondary metastasis blocking nodes and lymphatics, or from external compression.
- **Infection** with *Wucheria bancrofti* leading to fibrosis is the commonest cause worldwide and may lead to massive enlargement commonly called elephantiasis. Tuberculosis may also cause lymphoedema.
- **Radiation and surgery**, particularly of nodes, are important iatrogenic causes. Breast cancer surgery is the commonest cause in the developed world; 8% of patients will have lymphoedema that may be delayed in appearance for up to a year, and the risk increases with radiotherapy. It may also follow burns and burns surgery, and occasionally follows varicose vein stripping.

Investigation

Investigation often yields little information on the cause of the lymphoedema.

- Lymphangiography used to be the standard investigation but it has been largely replaced by less invasive techniques. A blue dye is injected into the first web space to reveal the lymphatics, which are subsequently injected with radio-opaque dye. It is tedious and time-consuming with some risk to the patient without actually providing information that would significantly change management. It may exacerbate the condition by inducing further fibrosis and valve damage.
  —Interstitial lymphangiography relies on the uptake of interstitial contrast by the lymphatics.
- Lymphoscintigraphy—technetium-labelled antimony injected intravenously is preferentially taken up by the lymphatics. This investigation is useful to define anatomy, patency and dynamics and is the standard investigation for lymphoedema.
- CT/MRI provide little extra information compared with lymphoscintigraphy. It can 'confirm' the diagnosis by demonstrating the classic honeycomb pattern with normal subfascial tissues, differentiating it from oedema and fat. It may be useful to rule out malignancy in selected cases.
- Doppler ultrasound can assess lymphatic and venous flow and is primarily used to exclude deep vein thrombosis.

Management

If possible, treat any treatable causes, e.g. diethylcarbamazine for early-stage filariasis (in later stages, when the worms die, they will still block the lymphatics).

Conservative
- Avoid standing for long periods of time
- Meticulous skin care to eradicate and prevent infection, especially of fungi
- Drug treatment
  —Antibiotics should be used to treat infections aggressively to minimize fibrosis. Long term use of antibiotics such as penicillins and cephalosporins may be used in recurrent cases.
  —Diuretics are generally contraindicated—there may be an improvement early on, but the effect is usually transient, and is counterproductive in the long run as the loss of interstitial fluid increases the protein concentration.
  —Benzopyrone can induce phagocytosis by binding to interstitial proteins, thus removing proteins, but clinical results have been mixed.

Physiotherapy
- Active physiological drainage (complex decongestive/regional physiotherapy) is applied in stages:
  —inpatient—'decongestive phase', that aims to massage lymph from the swelling toward healthy channels. This is followed by compressive bandaging and exercise
  —outpatient—support stockings and a regular exercise regime.

Surgical
Surgery is not the first option, and is used in only 10% of patients when conservative treatment fails. It is conventional to describe procedures as 'physiological' or 'excisional', but the distinction is not so clear-cut in practice, as 'physiological' procedures often have an excisional element as well.

- Physiological procedures aims to recreate working lymphatic channels but none are particularly successful and as such there is little to choose between the techniques. The long-term effects are unclear and largely unproven.
  —Lymphangioplasty—a variety of materials including silk sutures, teflon or rubber tubes have been implanted into the subcutaneous tissue in an effort to create drainage channels. It can be complicated by infection and extrusion, and long-term results are poor.
  —Pedicled omental transfer—in practice, the denuded mucosa of the omentum tends to be quickly surrounded by fibrosis rather than lymphatics and the long-term results are poor.
  —Enteromesenteric flap—a flap of ileum is used to cover transected lymph nodes.
  —Lymphovenous shunt (lymph node to vein or lymphatic to vein) may work better for early disease, particularly for genital lymphoedema.
  —Lympholymphatic anastomosis may be useful in cases where the disease is localized to a short segment, but is ineffective in those with hyperplastic disease.
- Excisional
  —Homans—(after Sistrunk) is the most popular surgical technique for lymphoedema. This is a staged excision of subcutaneous tissue and excess skin after 1-cm thick flaps are raised. The medial side is usually excised first with a second operation on the lateral side if required. Caution is required to avoid damage to

the common peroneal and sural nerves but the procedure is otherwise safe, reliable and produces consistent results.

—Charles—excision of lymphoedema and coverage with split skin grafts (occasionally full-thickness skin grafts) is usually reserved for extensive cases, particularly with ulceration. The results are aesthetically poor and the skin is unstable and prone to changes such as keratinization.

—Thomson—subcutaneous tissue is excised and a dermal flap is buried into the muscle compartment with the aim of merging dermal lymphatics with deep lymphatics. However, the results are generally poor and no definite connections have been demonstrated.

Liposuction has a temporary effect and requires repeating, and may actually cause further fibrosis. It may have a role as an adjunct to surgery in certain cases.

Further reading

Brennan MJ, Miller LT. Overview of treatment options and review of the current role and use of compression garments and exercise in the management of lymphoedema. *Cancer* 1998; **83:**2821–7.

Related topics of interest

- Liposuction
- Skin grafts.

Melanoma

Malignant melanomas (MMs) are neoplasms of the epidermal melanocytes that are derived embryologically from neural crest cells. Melanomas tend to affect younger patients with more females (2:1 in the US) compared with basal cell and squamous cell carcinomas. The lifetime risk of a Caucasian living in the UK is estimated to be approximately 1 in 80, but this increases five-fold if they emigrate to a sunnier climate such as Australia or South Africa.

Risk factors

- **Ultraviolet light**—sunlight, especially short, intense exposures resulting in sunburn as a child (before age 10) in the fair-skinned (Fitzpatrick type I), seems to be an important risk factor.
- **Xeroderma pigmentosa** is a rare sex-linked recessive disorder with faulty DNA repair, causing sunlight sensitivity. Many die from metastatic skin cancer.
- **Giant pigmented naevus** (20cm or 5% body surface area in size or greater). The varying reports in the literature quoting 10–40% incidence of malignant transformation of the lesion are probably overestimates; a figure of 5% derived from cancer registries is probably more accurate. Early excision of these lesions is generally recommended.
- **Dysplastic naevus syndrome** is a familial condition in which those affected have many (>100) small pigmented naevi (with lymphocytic infiltration). These patients have a 12× lifetime risk of malignant change, but prophylactic removal is not useful as the majority of melanomas arise de novo.
- **Familial melanoma** occurs in a small number of cases.

Historical subtypes

Various histological subtypes exist:

- **Superficial spreading MM** is the commonest subtype in Caucasians (70%) and often occurs on the legs in females and on the trunk in males. They are flat or slightly raised variegate lesions with a prolonged radial growth phase at the level of the epidermal–dermal junction before vertical growth leads to deeper invasion.
- **Nodular MM** (15–20%) forms typically blue–black nodules that may ulcerate or bleed with minor trauma. These are more common in males, whereas superficial spreading MM is more common in females.
- **Lentigo MM** (5–15%) appears as a brown macular patch with or without a discrete nodule, typically on the sun exposed areas i.e. head and neck or upper limbs of an elderly (F>M) patient. It has a prolonged radial growth phase and a better prognosis overall. Lentigo maligna (Hutchinson's freckle) is a precursor lesion (intraepithelial melanoma or in situ disease) and frank dermal invasion occurs in up to 30–50%; it should not be confused with lentigo simplex, which develops secondary to actinic damage and is very common with increasing age.

- **Acral lentiginous MM** is the most uncommon subtype in Caucasians but is more common (29–72% of all melanomas) in dark-skinned races. They can occur in the palms, soles, myocutaneous junctions or beneath the toe/finger nails (subungual MM, half involve the hallux).

Rare subtypes are amelanotic and desmoplastic melanomas.

Signs

The suspicious signs of a pigmented skin lesion are listed below:

ABCD

- **A**symmetry of lesion
- **B**order irregularity
- **C**olour—variegated, irregular brown–black colouring
- **D**iameter >6 mm.

also **E**levation/evolution/enlarging faster than other moles and **F**unny looking lesion

---

The criteria for diagnosis of MM are shown in Table 1.

Table 1 Criteria for diagnosis (Mackie).

Major criteria	Minor criteria (three or more)
Change in size (94%), shape (95%) or colour (89%). Without one major criteria, a lesion is unlikely to be a melanoma.	<ul><li>inflammation (51%)</li><li>bleeding/sensory change (46%)</li><li>crusting or oozing (31%)</li><li>diameter >7 mm</li></ul>

A **change** in a lesion is much more predictive than the absolute size.

Prognostic factors

Histological thickness is strongly related to prognosis; it can be measured in two different ways (see Table 2).

Table 2 Methods for measuring histological thickness.

Clark's levels (1969) describe the position of melanoma cells in the layers of skin	Breslow thickness (maximum distance from top of zona granulosa to base)
<ul><li>I. epidermis or carcinoma-in-situ</li><li>II. papillary dermis</li><li>III. up to papillary–reticular interface</li><li>IV. reticular dermis</li><li>V. subcutaneous tissue</li></ul>	<ul><li>thin—thickness of 0.75 mm or less</li><li>Intermediate——thickness of 0.76–1.50 mm——thickness of 1.51–4.00 mm</li><li>thick—thickness greater than 4.00 mm</li></ul>

The Breslow thickness is a better prognostic indicator and is easily reproducible between pathologists. Note, however, that it will tend to underestimate the thickness of ulcerated lesions.

The prognosis of melanoma is related to many factors including:

- **thickness** of lesion (most important, see Table 3)
- presence of lymph node metastases
- lesions with ulceration and high mitotic rate
- location—trunk lesions have a worse prognosis
- males and elderly patients fare less well.

Table 3 Lesion thickness and 5-year survival rates.

Thickness	Five-year survival rate
<0.76 mm	98–100%
>4 mm	47%

Staging

The AJCC melanoma staging system was officially changed in 2002 and there were several important differences from the old version:

- Tumour thickness is the predominant factor determining the T stage. The gradation is now more intuitive –1.0, 2.0 and 4.0 mm. The level of invasion (Clark's level) is important only in thin (T1) lesions. The presence of ulceration (which can be differentiated from traumatic loss of the surface) is a significant adverse prognostic factor.
- The number of, rather than the size of, lymph nodes, is important to the nodal stage. The tumour load in the nodes (micro- vs macro-metastasis) is also taken into account. Satellite lesions are considered together with in-transit lesions and is part of nodal disease (N2). The results of sentinel node biopsies are included.
- Lung metastases are considered separately from other types.

Investigations

- **Excisional biopsy**—A 2–5-mm margin is sufficient. Shave, punch or incisional biopsies are generally not recommended; the latter has theoretical issues with the potential implantation of tumour cells deeper and does not provide a complete picture of the depth of the lesion. Incisional biopsy may have a role in the assessment of larger lentigines. Reconstruction of the defect can be delayed until the final histology is known.
- **Secondary surgery**—subsequent excision margins are dictated by the thickness of the melanoma on histological sectioning. There are various guidelines available; UK guidelines suggest:

—Thin (<1 mm)	1 cm margin
—Intermediate (1–4 mm)	2 cm margin
—Thick (>4 mm)	Wider margins may be warranted to optimize local control, but do not impact on the overall survival. Overall there are little data to support the usefulness of a wide excision margin.

American guidelines (2002 AJCC) are:
 —0–1 mm   1 cm margin
 —1–2 mm   2 cm margin
 —>2 mm   2 cm margin

(Balch et al. 2001)

- Thin melanomas need no further investigation, whereas thicker melanomas should be staged by contrast CT (chest, abdomen and pelvis), USG abdomen, chest X-ray (CXR) and liver function tests (LFTs).
- There is no adjunctive treatment of proven benefit, but there are several clinical trials investigating the role of interferons and anti-GM2. Interferons are licensed for use as an adjunctive treatment but are awaiting 'recommendation'.

Management of lymph nodes

Clinically palpable lymph nodes are investigated with FNA or biopsy, and if found to be positive, then a block dissection is offered. There is some controversy with regards to the extent of the en bloc dissections, especially in the groin. Wound problems and postoperative lymphoedema are not uncommon (25%).

Clinically impalpable nodes are more difficult to deal with:

- Surgery is not indicated for thin lesions (<1 mm) because the yield is low—the risk of metastasis is nearly 0%; only 5–10% will have occult nodes.
- Conversely, elective node surgery will be of little use in thick lesions (>4 mm) because of the high chance of occult distant metastasis (66%) and elective surgery has no effect on prognosis, although it may offer better local control.
- In intermediate thickness lesions the risk of metastasis is 50%:
  —**Elective lymph node dissection** (ELND, Balch) may theoretically be useful but has not been shown to provide any survival benefit and is generally not performed except within the context of a trial.
  —**Sentinel node biopsy** (SNB)—the rationale is that lymph flows predictably to a sentinel node first. If this node can be detected and sampled, then subsequent treatment can be based on this. However, there is no evidence to suggest that SNB affects prognosis.
    —Preoperative formal lymphoscintigraphy is performed after a radioisotope is injected intradermally to the scar or lesion if it has not already been removed. It may identify in-transit lesions or the nodal groups likely to drain lymph from the melanoma.
    —Perioperative injection of blue dye and/or radioisotope (technetium) labelled colloid. After 20 min the 'hot' blue node is found and resected.
    —There is much debate concerning frozen sections; they are not recommended in many studies because they only have a sensitivity of 50–60%; instead, formal 'paraffin' sections and immunohistochemistry are preferable as they increase detection. Sensitivity can be increased further by using tyrosinase PCR.

Further reading

Balch CM, Buzaid AC, Soong SJ et al. Final version of the American Joint Committee on Cancer staging system for cutaneous melanoma. *J Clin Oncol* 2001; **19:**3635–3648.

Murray CS, Stockton DL, Doherty VR. Thick melanoma: the challenge persists. *Br J Dermatol* 2005; **152:**104–9.

Related topic of interest

- Ultraviolet light.

Microsurgery and tissue transfer

Microsurgical free tissue transfer allows tissue to be transferred from one part of the body to another and allows for its immediate vascularization. This enables reconstruction and wound closure to be achieved where grafts would not be a viable option, e.g. when covering bare bone or tendon. 'Free' flaps are distinguished from local and pedicle flaps that remain attached to the body and their blood supply during positional transfer. The anastomosis of blood vessels, an artery and vein, can require specialized techniques and instruments and a prolonged anaesthetic. Nevertheless, in experienced hands, microsurgical free tissue transfer has a high rate of success, in the region of 95–99%. The technique is particularly useful in the following conditions:

- stable coverage of exposed vital structures, e.g. in complex tibial fractures
- vascularized bone, e.g. for mandible reconstruction
- functional tissue, e.g. muscle for facial reanimation
- bulky soft tissue, e.g. breast reconstruction or to obliterate cavities.

Care needs to be taken in patients who have undergone previous irradiation or are smokers. Nicotine affects the microcirculation and wound healing—the rate of partial muscle necrosis is doubled and skin loss and infection (30%) is increased. Overall, smoker status does not affect the rate of total flap loss, suggesting that the anastomosis itself is not threatened. Smokers should be advised not to smoke for at least two weeks before and after surgery.

Decision making is as critical to the success of flap microsurgery as surgical technique. The choice of flap should be appropriate to the problem, with alternatives in mind should it fail.

- The recipient vessel should be out of the zone of injury or irradiation. Doppler ultrasound may be useful to detect suitable vessels.
- Anastomosis requires meticulous technique; in particular limiting unnecessary manipulation of the vessels. The adventitia is trimmed and the vessel ends sutured without excess tension using 8-0 to 11-0 non-absorbable monofilament sutures. End-to-side anastomosis is useful when there is a significant size discrepancy—it is as effective as end-to-end anastomosis. Alternatives to sutures include devices such as couplers and staples, but these are not in common use.
- Vein grafts may be needed when there is insufficient vessel length. The length of the vein graft does not seem to affect patency per se, but increasing the length increases the risk of thrombosis and kinking. Diameter discrepancies of more than a factor of two should be avoided, otherwise there is an increased risk of turbulent flow and thrombosis.

Postoperative management

Regular flap observations are important. The 'window' for rescuing a flap is rather narrow, especially for muscle flaps, which can be compromised very quickly and may also cause systemic upset. Preferably, the patient should be monitored in a 'flap ward' with experienced staff and where ambient temperatures can be controlled. Clinically, a combination of colour, capillary refill (1–2 s), temperature and turgor is used to assess the state of the flap. Careful puncture (avoiding the pedicle!) or scratching with a needle-tip to assess bleeding may also be used.

Some advocate more objective measurements for flap monitoring:

- Temperature probes—a flap–core temperature difference of more than 2°C suggests a perfusion problem.
- Laser Doppler techniques measure blood flow but only penetrate 1.5 mm; near-infrared spectroscopy is similar but has better penetration.
- Surface Doppler (may record false-positives by picking up other vessels).
- Pulse oximetry, particularly for replanted digits.
- IV fluorescein and a Woods lamp.

However, none of these show demonstrable superiority over combined clinical assessment.

The patient should be kept 'well, warm and wet'.

- **Well.** Give adequate analgesia to prevent pain and anxiety, which can lead to vasoconstriction.
- **Warm.** Keep the flap (and the patient) warm.
- **Wet.** Hyperdynamic circulation (systolic blood pressure >100 mmHg) is maintained to maximize perfusion through the anastomosis. Intravenous fluid is given to maintain a urine output of at least 1 ml/kg/h.
- Anticoagulation, e.g. Dextran 40 at 20 ml/h for 5 days is used by some to reduce platelet adhesiveness. Alternatives include heparin (reduces platelet aggregation) or aspirin. There is no evidence of usefulness in uncomplicated anastomosis and there is a risk of haematoma formation or anaphylaxis.
- Elevate flap area where possible to reduce swelling and promote venous drainage.

Potential problems

A free flap may be compromised by inflow or outflow problems.

- Arterial problems—cool pale flap with sluggish capillary refill
- Venous problems—blue congested flap with brisk refill.

Simple measures may be useful:

- Assess and optimize hydration
- Reposition patient
- Remove constricting dressings or tight sutures.

But if unsuccessful, re-exploration is required and has a 75% success rate on average.

- Optimize the patient's haemodynamics.
- Consider applying antispasmodics such as lignocaine, papaverine or verapamil to the vessel.
- Check for twisting of the vessels or anastomosis.
- Re-do the anastomosis if necessary.

- Antifibrinolytics such as streptokinase or TPA may be useful, but there is a risk of haemorrhage.
- Anticoagulants may be useful postoperatively.

Flaps may be damaged by **reperfusion injury**: anaerobic metabolites build up in ischaemic tissue and on re-establishing blood flow, oxygen free radicals are generated causing calcium influx and cell damage. **'No reflow'** describes the situation of having no flow despite a physically patent anastomosis; this has been attributed to platelet aggregation, endothelial injury and fluid shift into tissues (from failing cellular pumps).

Failing flaps
- Leeches (from the Old English 'laece' for physician) are useful for cases of venous congestion. The leech itself (*Hirudo medicinalis*) sucks around 10 ml of blood, but in addition, the hirudin in its saliva is a selective thrombin inhibitor and will promote another 50 ml of loss through oozing. Substantial blood loss may require transfusion. Prophylaxis (augmentin) against *Aeromonas hydrophilus* is needed.
- Hyperbaric oxygen (HBO) has been shown to be useful for salvaging failing flaps in some animal studies, but there is little clinical data on its role. Use is infrequent because it requires access to an HBO facility and can be costly. Complications are rare but it may cause seizures due to oxygen toxicity and barotraumas to the middle ear and pneumothorax.

Further reading

Whitaker IS, Izadi D, Oliver DW et al. *Hirudo medicinalis* and the plastic surgeon. *Br J Plast Surg* 2004; **57:**348–53.

Related topic of interest

- Breast reconstruction.

Neck dissection

If malignant cells from head and neck cancer spread into lymphatic channels and cause metastatic neck disease, there is a great negative impact on the survival of the patient. Successful management of metastatic neck disease is extremely important.

Assessment

History and examination is vital.

- Clinical assessment by palpation alone is not wholly reliable, with a false-negative rate of one-third in especially short fat necks or after radiotherapy.
- Ultrasound scan with fine-needle-aspiration cytology has high specificity but sensitivity is an issue.
- CT can demonstrate features suggesting malignancy, including central necrosis, capsule enhancement and extracapsular spread.
- MRI is more sensitive and will demonstrate more nodes, but is less able to differentiate benign or reactive nodes from malignant nodes.

Levels of the neck nodes

A significant advance in the discussion and comparison of neck disease and its treatment was the use of a consistent nomenclature (Memorial Sloan-Kettering), as described in Table 1.

- Nx not assessable
- N0 no nodes
- N1 single ipsilateral, 3 cm or less
- N2a single ipsilateral, >3 cm, <6 cm
- N2b multiple ipsilateral, <6 cm
- N2c bilateral/contralateral <6 cm
- N3 massive >6 cm.

The prognosis is significantly worse if the nodes show fixity, extracapsular spread, perivascular or perineural invasion, or if they occur in the posterior triangle or contralateral neck.

Surgical management

A neck dissection (ND) is effectively a block dissection of the regional lymphatic system:

- **Radical**—a radical ND aims to remove the contents of the first five nodal levels, from mandible to clavicle, and from lateral sternohyoid to anterior trapezius.
- **Extended** ND—as above, but with additional structures such as the paratracheal, retropharyngeal and mediastinal nodes, and the parotid gland.

Table 1 Classification of lymph nodes of the neck.

Node level	Name	Boundaries	Comments
I	Submandibular triangle	Between lower mandible border and bellies of digastric muscles	Ia submental triangle Ib digastric triangle
II	Upper jugular	From base of skull to carotid bifurcation	Jugulodigastric node drains oral cavity, face and scalp IIa anterior to accessory IIb posterior to accessory
III	Middle jugular	From carotid bifurcation to the omohyoid	
IV	Lower jugular	From the omohyoid to the clavicle	Contains the thoracic duct
V	Posterior triangle	Posterior border sternomastoid, anterior trapezius and clavicle	Cervical plexus Transverse cervical artery
VI	Anterior compartment	Hyoid to suprasternal notch, between lateral borders of sternohyoid	A later addition to the original scheme

- **Modified radical** ND—as above, but sparing one or more non-lymphatic structures.
- **Selective**—one or more node groups is spared, i.e. subtotal.

Radical neck dissection

Radical neck dissection (RND, Crile 1906) removes the nodal contents plus non-lymphatic structures such as the accessory nerve, sternomastoid and internal jugular vein. The morbidity of the procedure is mainly related to the excision of the non-lymphatic structures:

- **Spinal accessory**—possible problems include discomfort and reduced abduction, asymmetry of neck outline and drooping shoulder.
- **Internal jugular vein** (IJV)—it is reported that bilateral RND results in an increase in intracranial pressure with an increased risk of stroke and blindness. The mortality of bilateral RND is said to be 10–14% compared to 0–3% in unilateral surgery. Generally, it is recommended that bilateral operations should be staged, or the internal jugular vein should be reconstructed with greater saphenous vein, for example.
- **Sternomastoid**—the removal of this muscle has the least associated morbidity; the problem is mainly a cosmetic issue, although it can offer protection for the carotid sheath.

Table 2 explains when RND should be considered.

Table 2 Indications and contraindications for radical neck dissection.

Indications for RND	Contraindications of RND
• High-grade tumours with N2 neck • Recurrent disease • Invasive nodal disease—extracapsular spread, involving IJV or accessory • Postradiotherapy, if the primary is under control.	• Uncontrollable primary • N0 neck • Metastasis • Fixed neck/encased carotid.

Modified radical neck dissection

Modified radical neck dissection (MRND) was designed in an effort to reduce the morbidity by preserving one or more non-lymphatic functional structures when onco-logically safe to do so. There is a classification described by Medina:

• type 1—accessory nerve preserved
• type 2—accessory nerve and sternomastoid preserved
• type 3—all three (accessory nerve, sternomastoid and IJV) preserved.

The actual type of dissection is often decided perioperatively according to the find-ings. An MRND is the operation of choice in most cases, except where RND is specif-ically indicated. Outcomes in selected cases are similar, but there are no prospective studies comparing RND and MRND. Studies that do exist suffer from the fact that many preceded the standardized classification of neck dissections.

Selective neck dissection

From a review of surgical specimens at the Sloan-Kettering hospital, it was found that nodal spread is largely predictable, in that it follows certain characteristic and consis-tent patterns. This led to the development of the concept of the selective neck dissec-tion with the aim of clearing levels most likely to be involved and to avoid unnecessary additional morbidity, as explained in Table 3. It often serves the purpose of a staging procedure.

Adjunctive radiotherapy

Postoperative radiotherapy may be indicated for:

• positive histology on neck dissection specimens
• extracapsular spread
• N2 disease.

Table 3 Classification of selective neck dissection.

Selective neck dissection	Levels resected	Indications	Comments
Supraomohyoid	Levels 1, 2 and 3	For oral cancer. Can be viewed as essentially being a staging procedure	Spares thoracic duct, accessory nerve, sternomastoid and IJV. Not suitable for tonsillar tumours
Anterolateral	Levels 2, 3 and 4	For laryngeal and hypopharyngeal cancers	
Anterior	Levels 2, 3, 4 and tracheo-oesophageal nodes	For thyroid cancers	
Posterior	Levels 2, 3, 4 and 5	Posterior scalp cancers	

Complications of neck dissection

General discussions of complications should be divided into specific and general, immediate or operative, early, intermediate or late. There are some specific complications worthy of mention:

- Lymph/chyle leak due to damage of the thoracic duct (left neck). It can usually be managed conservatively
  —low-fat diet
  —total parenteral nutrition can significantly reduce the volume of leakage within 24 h
  —electrolytes need to be monitored carefully.
- Salivary fistula
- Nerve damage causing difficulty swallowing (glossopharyngeal), shoulder pain and weakness (XI), difficulty breathing (phrenic—a raised hemidiaphragm is seen on chest radiographs) and tongue weakness (hypoglossal). Trigger point sensitivity may be due to neuroma formation
- Skin flap necrosis—care needs to be taken when this occurs over the great vessels.

Skin incisions

There are a significant number of different neck incision lines. The general principles that are common to them all are:

- Try to place incisions along relaxed skin tension lines. Contracture can be reduced by careful design of the incision lines, e.g. right angles and lazy 'S's.
- Submandibular incisions should be at least 2 cm below the level of the mandible to avoid damaging the marginal mandibular branch of the facial nerve.

- Be wary of incisions in the watershed areas of blood supply; Y-incisions should not be placed over the carotid artery.
- Skin flaps should be raised in the subplatysmal if it is possible and not oncologically unsafe.

Specific incisions

- **McFee**—double neck incisions, one above and one below (at least 7 cm apart). Cosmesis is good and the flaps have a good blood supply and so this incision is suited to provide reliable coverage of the great vessels in postradiotherapy necks. However, there is a steeper learning curve—dissection is more tedious and difficult due to limited exposure.
- **Y-incision (Conley)**—the curved vertical limb decreases the risk of scar contracture. There is excellent exposure of the neck but there is a risk of flap necrosis exposing vessels, making it a dangerous option in the postradiotherapy neck.
- **Schobinger**—high horizontal incision with posterior vertical limb allows easier access to the oral cavity in particular.
- **Hockey stick**—mastoid to shoulder.
- **Apron**—mastoid to symphysis (unilateral), mastoid to mastoid (bilateral).

Further reading

Divvuri U, Simental AA Jr, D'Angelo G et al. Elective neck dissection and survival in patients with squamous cell carcinoma of the oral cavity and oropharynx. *Laryngoscope* 2004; **114:**2228–34.

Necrotizing fasciitis

Necrotizing fasciitis (NF) is a rapidly progressive soft tissue infection with widespread fascial necrosis and secondary necrosis of the superficial tissues as a result of vascular occlusion. Bacterial spread along fascial planes is facilitated by bacterial enzymes and toxins (haemolysins, hyaluronidase, streptokinase, etc.).

The onset of this disease is usually insidious, initially the patient may seem deceptively well with only flu-like constitutional upset with fevers and chills. However it can progress rather quickly.

- Disproportionate and extreme pain changes to anaesthesia as the superficial nerves are damaged.
- Initial spreading erythema darkens to purple and grey-duskiness. Multiple areas may appear to coalesce into one large area. Swelling with vesicles, blisters and bullae may form. Crepitus may be present, especially in diabetics.
- Extreme toxicity and septicaemia develops.

The mortality rate is high (25–50% is commonly quoted). Mortality is highest in those with delayed debridement, the elderly and those with diabetes mellitus. NF can affect all areas; Fournier's gangrene is a subset that is localized to the scrotum/perineum and typically is idiopathic with 75% mortality.

Although NF may be found in the immunosuppressed (HIV, cancer, diabetes and in transplant patients):

- Half of patients were previously fit and well.
- It can develop after relatively minor trauma, insect bites, surgery (such as drainage of intraperitoneal or perianal/ischiorectal abscesses) or even needle puncture, such as intramuscular or intravenous injections.

Intravenous drugs users are at risk of NF from anaerobic streptococci, whereas those with liver disease are susceptible to *Vibrio vulnificus* from raw seafood, especially oysters, which often causes haemorrhagic blisters.

NF is a rather general term to describe soft tissue infections involving the fascia that may have many causes. There are three main types, and distinguishing between them is useful as the optimal treatment is significantly different in each case.

1. **Polymicrobial**—this is the commonest type. There is synergy between anaerobes and facultative aerobes, especially gram negatives. The organisms are able to proliferate in the local tissue hypoxia that develops after tissue injury secondary to trauma or surgery, particularly in the unwell. Hypoxia reduces neutrophil function that facilitates bacterial growth.
2. **Streptococcal** (group A) aka 'the flesh eating bug'—the streptococcal pyrogenic exotoxins (SPE) and streptococcal superantigen (SSA) are directly toxic. The injury may be quite minor; the overlying skin may look viable despite extensive underlying necrosis. Streptococci and sometimes staphylococci are the initiators, but other organisms may be present such as *Bacteroides* and *Escherichia coli*, and may contribute by reducing phagocytic function and interferon secretion. Gas may be present but is not a common feature. This form of NF has a worse prognosis and

is more rapidly progressive. There is an unexplained association with the use of non-steroidal anti-inflammatory agents such as ibuprofen during zoster infection.

3. **Clostridial myonecrosis**/gas gangrene can happen after trauma/surgery (*Clostridium perfringens*) or spontaneously (*Clostridium septicum*). Gas and crepitus is a characteristic feature. Septicum infection may be associated with colonic carcinoma and leukaemia.

Investigations

- Blood tests may typically show a raised white cell count and a low plasma sodium level.
- Fluid wound aspirate for gram stain.
- Rapid streptococcal diagnosis can be obtained by PCR of the SPE genes.
- Radiography is generally uninformative unless there is gas, but gas is not specific to clostridia. It may also be seen in infections of *Bacteroides*, *E. coli*, or *Peptococcus*; hydrogen, nitrogen and hydrogen sulphide are produced.
- CT may be useful to establish the extent of the necrosis and is more sensitive in detecting gas, but is generally non-specific. MRI can detect fascial necrosis.
- **Biopsy** is important. It gathers material for culture, gram staining and histology (necrosis with thrombi in occluded vessels). It is important to biopsy either the periphery or the deep margin, because central parts may have bacteria that do not actually contribute to the process. A microbiology opinion is advisable.

Treatment

Aggressive resuscitation with fluids and oxygen is needed. **High-dose antibiotics** are administered depending on the gram stain results. Empiric treatment (e.g. gentamycin, clindamycin with or without ampicillin) can be commenced until definitive results are available.

- Aerobes are mostly gram negatives (ampicillin and gentamicin)
- Anaerobes (metronidazole, clindamycin or a third-generation cephalosporin such as ceftriaxone)
- Streptococcal (penicillin G or clindamycin)
  —Clindamycin is said to destroy the toxin SPE.

Immediate aggressive debridement of the necrosis down to viable tissue is important. Muscle is often healthy underneath the necrotic fascia. The wound is left open and evaluated daily in the operating theatre.

Hyperbaric oxygen (HBO) may be an option after antibiotics and surgery. It may reduce spreading and improve tissue perfusion, but there are no randomized trials confirming its usefulness.

Further reading

Bachmeyer C, Langman B, Blum L. Fulminant streptococcal necrotizing fasciitis. *Dermatology* 2004; **209:**346–7.

Neurofibromatosis

Neurofibromatoses are multisystem genetic disorders that can be classified as hamartoses. There are two subtypes, which are actually different diseases:

- **Neurofibromatosis type 1** (NF1)—'typical' multiple cutaneous lesions. The overall prognosis is better than for type 2 due to a lower risk of central nervous system (CNS) tumours.
- **Neurofibromatosis type 2** (NF2)—the primary features are the vestibular schwannomas and other CNS/spinal tumours such as meningiomas. Hearing loss is the commonest presentation.

Neurofibromatosis type 1 (von Recklinghausen's disease)

There is a mutation on the NF1 gene on chromosome 17. The gene product is neurofibromin, a tumour suppressor whose precise role is unclear, but it has diverse functions as demonstrated by the myriad of manifestations. The defect can be detected only in two-thirds of the 'clinically affected'; prenatal diagnosis is possible but is not widely available.

NF1 occurs in approximately 1 in 3000 people, with approximately half being new cases due to de novo mutations. It is inherited in an autosomal dominant manner; penetrance is near complete but with very variable manifestations. Patients may have short stature, scoliosis, macrocephaly and have learning difficulties with or without attention deficit (40%) but patients generally lead productive lives. There is no predilection for gender or race. Life expectancy may be reduced by around 15 years, due to:

- hypertension that is usually 'essential'; but there is an increased frequency of phaeochromocytomas and renal vascular stenoses
- spinal cord lesions. Dumbbell tumours may require surgery
- tumours. Benign (neurofibromas and gliomas) and malignant (neurosarcoma).

The features tend to appear gradually and if an 'at risk' individual does not develop any typical features by the age of 10, then they are judged to be unaffected. A positive diagnosis is made if a patient has two or more of the following features:

- First-degree relative with the disease.
- Six or more café au lait spots of 5 mm or more in those less than 10 years of age, or 15 mm or more in an adult. This is often the first finding. The spots tend to fade with age and the response to laser treatment is variable.
- Optic nerve gliomas typically present as visual loss before the age of 5 years, but tend not to be as progressive as gliomas in non-neurofibromatosis patients.
- Axillary and inguinal freckles generally appear later in childhood.
- Lisch nodules (iris hamartomas).
- Two or more typical neurofibromas, or one plexiform neurofibroma. The typical neurofibromas appear around puberty and are generally well-differentiated lesions that undergo malignant transformation to sarcomas only occasionally. Plexiform neurofibromas usually appear at an earlier age in children and tend to be diffuse and locally 'invasive'. They may cause pain or bone erosion. These lesions may require excision but seem to have more wound healing problems subsequently.

- Sphenoid dysplasia (usually asymptomatic). And other bony abnormalities such as intramedullary fibrosis and cortical thinning. Long bone abnormalities such as bowing of the tibia due to pseudoarthroses—this commonly leads to amputation, but this is less frequent.

Investigations

CT/MRI should not be used routinely but only for selected indications, e.g. CNS lesions and optic nerve problems. Slit lamp examination for Lisch nodules is useful for screening family members.

Neurofibromatosis type 2

This is a less common disorder and shows autosomal dominant inheritance with high penetrance. The defect lies on a different chromosome—a deletion on chromosome number 22; a direct gene test is available. The commonest lesion is a schwannoma; true neurofibromas are actually rare, and hence some propose the alternative terms, schwannomatosis or MISME (multiple inherited schwannomas, meningiomas and ependymomas).

Most diagnoses are made before age 40 and 45% present with hearing loss, tinnitus or balance problems in their 30s (the spontaneous form of vestibular schwannomas tends to occur later in life). These tumours are often erroneously called 'acoustic neuromas'; they are more likely to encase the facial and vestibulocochlear cranial nerves, making them more likely to be symptomatic at a relatively small size and making resection more difficult. Presentation as a child is less common but may occur due to ocular abnormalities. Most patients require at least one operation in their lifetimes; radiotherapy is an option if surgery is not possible.

The diagnosis is made from either:

- bilateral vestibulocochlear schwannoma on CT/MRI. Biopsy is not required, or
- first-degree relative and:
  —early-onset vestibulocochlear schwannoma or
  —any two of the following: meningioma (often multiple and affects the thoracic spine), glioma, schwannoma (may be cutaneous) and juvenile posterior subcapsular lenticular opacity/cataracts.

The finding of any cranial nerve schwannoma should prompt screening; any cranial nerve from the oculomotor to the hypoglossal can be involved, with the vestibulocochlear and trigeminal nerves most commonly being involved. Malignant transformation is rare (less than 1%).

MRI is the examination of choice, providing superior imaging and characterization to CT—typically the lesion is mushroom or ice-cream cone shaped. Necrosis may be seen as tumours enlarge.

Further reading

Arun D, Gietman DH. Recent advances in neurofibromatosis type 1. *Curr Opin Neurol* 2004; **17**:101–5.

Related topic of interest

- Facial reanimation.

Oral cancer

The oral cavity starts at the lips and ends at the line marked by the junction of the hard and soft palates and the circumvallate papillae. It has an important role in swallowing, taste and speech.

Head and neck cancers constitute 15% of all cancers, and one-third of all head and neck tumours arise within the oral cavity. The vast majority of oral cancers are squamous cell carcinomas (SCC, 90%); adenocarcinomas are the second commonest, while other types of tumour are fairly uncommon. The patient (males predominate 3–4×) usually presents with a painless ulcer or cervical lymphadenopathy.

The risk factors (for SCC) are usually summarized as the 'S's, and of these **smoking** is the most important. Those who do not give up smoking have a greater risk of recurrence and of developing a second primary SCC. Chewing tobacco or betel nuts also increases risk. Susceptibility to these factors may be at least partly determined by genetic factors. The other 'S's are **spirits** (the effect of alcohol and tobacco is additive, and both show a linear association with cancer risk), **sharps** (damaged teeth or ill-fitting dental appliances), and less commonly, **syphilis** and **spices**. Leukoplakia and erythroplakia are premalignant lesions that are found in association with up to 20% of oral cancers; these lesions can progress to frankly invasive SCC and such lesions tend to be more aggressive.

Specific areas

Tongue (20–30% of oral cancers. Of these lesions 75% or more occur on the anterior portion). Tumour depth has been shown to be predictive of neck node involvement and thus elective nodal dissection is recommended by some for lesions thicker than 10 mm. Over one-third of lesions will have occult nodes even for early tumours.

Floor of the mouth (30–35%, but 50% or more in Indians due to betel nut chewing). One-fifth of T1 tumours have occult neck nodes and overall 30% have nodes at presentation.

The **retromolar trigone** is the area behind the lower third molar tooth. Tumours here will drain to the jugulodigastric node and submandibular area. Early bone involvement is common, as is spread into nearby structures such as nerve infiltration and muscle involvement causing trismus. Lesions of the tonsils behave similarly but rarely involve bone.

Assessment

History taking and a thorough systematic examination of the whole oral cavity, including a bimanual examination, will provide a diagnosis in 90% of cases.

Specific investigation includes:

- Tissue diagnosis is provided by biopsy of lesions along with panendoscopy, which is essential to exclude synchronous tumours (i.e. within 6 months, otherwise called metachronous) that occur in 5–15% of patients in the oesophagus, oropharynx and lung.

- Fine-needle aspiration (FNA) of any neck masses; tongue and floor of mouth tumours will have nodes in 30–40% at presentation.
- Imaging with MRI and CT is useful to define the extent of the tumour. Tissue characterization is generally better with MRI; it is more reliable for detecting lymph nodes and extracapsular spread in nodes less than 2cm in size. CT is supposedly better for determining cortical bone involvement and malignant nodes. Orthopantomograms may also provide useful information. The periosteum is not a wholly reliable barrier to tumour spread, particularly after radiotherapy.

The most widely accepted method of defining the extent of the disease is TNM (tumour node metastasis) staging (see also Table 1).

Tis in situ cancer	N1 single ipsilateral mobile node less
T1 2cm or less	than 3cm
T2 more than 2cm but not more	N2a single ipsilateral node 3–6cm
than 4cm	N2b multiple ipsilateral less than 6cm
T3 more than 4cm	N2c bilateral/contralateral less than 6cm
T4 more than 4cm and invasion	N3 fixed, multiple nodes more than 6cm
of adjacent structures	
including bone	

Table 1 Staging of oral cancers and associated survival rates.

Stage	TNM	Survival
Stage I	T1N0M0	90%
Stage II	T2N0M0	50–70%
Stage III	T3 or T(1–3)N1	40%
Stage IV	T4 or N2/N3 or M1	25%

Treatment

For Stage I or II tumours, either surgery or radiotherapy alone works well. The choice is related to patient preference and local expertise. For persistent or recurrent disease the other modality is still available. For more advanced tumours, surgery and radiotherapy are combined, but response is generally poor.

Surgery should be radical where possible to improve survival. Gross margins of 1–2cm should be taken and frozen-section analysis of the resection margins is recommended. The propensity for perineural spread along the lingual and inferior alveolar nerve means that these should be divided higher up if possible. Surgery debulks most of the tumour (>99%) and provides staging information; radiotherapy is still available as a 'back-up' if excision margins are involved.

Radiotherapy in the form of external beam irradiation with or without internal radiotherapy (brachytherapy) is as effective as surgery for small lesions. Radiotherapy can retain function to a greater extent than surgery can, and the neck can be treated at the same time. Contraindications for radiotherapy include previous radiotherapy, close proximity to bone and those with known poor healing. Treatment causes xerostomia, decreased taste and mucositis, all of which may lead to reduced feeding and weight loss.

The role of chemotherapy as a primary treatment is unclear, and this situation is not helped by the lack of standard protocols. However, as an adjunct, there is definitive evidence of its usefulness.

- Neoadjuvant or induction chemotherapy aims to decrease the size of massive tumours, which may then become operable.
- Consolidation chemotherapy can be utilized after surgery for advanced tumours.

Intra-arterial (IA) chemotherapy aims to deliver a large localized dose to the tumour area; it is typically given as four weekly doses with concurrent radiotherapy. Its usefulness has not been fully determined.

Nodal disease
Treatment of neck disease may be:

- therapeutic—i.e. to treat detectable nodal disease. Neck dissection and irradiation are both effective.
- prophylactic—i.e. clinically no cervical neck nodes.

When the neck is not clinically involved (N0 neck), there is a choice: to keep the situation under observation (not generally advocated as even for T1/2 lesions there is a significant risk of occult nodal involvement) or to perform a supraomohyoid (selective) neck dissection, and then if two or more nodes are involved, adjuvant radiotherapy can be given. The choice of initial radiation or surgery depends on the treatment mode of the primary, patient preference and health and local facilities.

The method of reconstruction depends upon the extent of resection.

- Direct closure or even healing by second intention is suitable for small defects in certain areas, e.g. buccal mucosa, floor of the mouth.
- Skin grafts are simple and reliable, but can contract and so cause tethering, and may be no better than the above in the long term for small lesions. They may be suitable for large superficial defects such as those of the hard palate. Fenestration and quilting are preferred to the use of tie-over dressings.
- Local (mucosal) flaps such as the tongue and buccal mucosa are used less. The nasolabial flap can provide reliable though small pieces (6×3 cm) of tissue and requires two stages. The temporalis may also be suitable for small volumes and can be raised as muscle or fascial flaps; the donor is reasonably well hidden but requires rather extensive dissection with a small risk of damaging the facial nerve.
- Larger volumes of tissue transfer require pedicled flaps such as the deltopectoral, latissimus doris and pectoralis major flaps. The pectoralis major flap is very reliable and can be raised with a rib segment, but requires a large amount of dissection and the donor is not aesthetic, particularly in females. In addition, there is a bulky tunnel in the neck and the flap itself is usually too bulky for the tongue and floor of the mouth (and may also have hairs).
- Free flaps can be used depending on the requirements:
  —For bulk, e.g. muscle, the rectus femoris is particularly useful.

—For coverage, then thin fascial flaps such as the radial forearm free flap (RFFF), lateral arm flap or anterolateral thigh flap are better. The RFFF is thin, pliable and reliable, and can be raised with the brachioradialis. In addition, a two-team approach can be used; however, the donor often needs skin grafting. The lateral arm flap is similar to the RFFF but the vascular pedicle is more variable.

Further reading

Nicoletti G, Soutar DS, Jackson MS et al. Chewing and swallowing after surgical treatment for oral cancer: functional evaluation in 196 selected cases. *Plast Reconstr Surg* 2004; **114:**329–38.

Related topics of interest

- Neck dissection
- Premalignant lesions.

Paediatric burns

Children's burns are commonly caused by accidents and more than 60% are scalds. The group most at risk comprises males in their second year of life: they have the physical capability to explore their environment but lack the awareness of its dangers.

There are significant characteristics that distinguish the paediatric burn and its management from the same burn in an adult.

Acute care (ABC)

- **Airway**—as the airway of a child is narrower and more irritable, it is more prone to obstruction: any degree of swelling is going to have a relatively greater obstructive effect.
- **Breathing**—children are more reliant on diaphragmatic breathing. Inhalational injuries may have prolonged adverse effects on the respiratory function.
- **Circulation**—intravenous access may be difficult due to the vessel size and the amount of subcutaneous fat: options for access include the femoral vein, a cut-down of the long saphenous vein or an intra-osseus line. Blood pressure is generally well maintained even with severe hypovolaemia; overt shock is generally a late feature.

Depth of burn

The thickness of a child's skin significantly influences the depth of burn sustained by a given injury. A given trauma will cause deeper burns in an infant compared to adults, because of their thinner skin. Water at 60°C will cause a full-thickness burn in:

- less than 1s in an infant
- 20s in an adult.

Burn depth, particularly after scalds, is generally more difficult to judge in children. They are often 'mixed depth' and can develop further over 48h. Laser Doppler imaging may provide more accurate objective measures of burn depth but requires specialized equipment; an alternative is the selective use of test shaves under anaesthesia, which may help to identify those most likely to benefit from surgery. Often it is better to give them 'the benefit of the doubt' for 10–14 days before embarking on surgery.

Surface area

Due to the different body proportions in children, Wallace's rule of nines in its basic form cannot be applied; it can be modified to take account of the patient's age.

- from birth up to 1 year of age, the surface area of the head and neck is 18% and for the leg it is 14%
- for each year after, the head loses 1% and each leg gains 0.5%
- and so by 10 years, the adult proportions are attained.

The formula becomes rather unwieldy, and it is preferable to use a Lund and Browder burns chart.

Children have a greater surface area:volume ratio than adults and this has several effects:

- increases metabolic rate—care and attention needs to be paid to providing adequate calories in large burns. The Galveston formula is one way of calculating the nutritional requirements; the Curreri formula can be used in both children and adults
- increases heat loss (less fat and shivering)—child should be kept warm and the ambient temperature should be raised if necessary
- increases evaporative water loss.

Resuscitation

The Parklands formula is a suitable guide for the resuscitation of paediatric burn patients, but maintenance fluids also need to be given (see Table 1).

Table 1   Fluids in paediatric burns.

Resuscitation	Maintenance
2–4 × burn surface area (%) × body weight (kg)	100 ml per kg for the first 10 kg 50 ml per kg for the next 10 kg 20 ml per kg for the rest
Lower threshold: 10% burn	
Ringer's lactate	Dextrose water

Fluid administration should be adjusted to maintain urine output at 1 ml/kg/h or more. The renal tubules have a reduced capacity to concentrate urine, hence urine output tends to be maintained even when the volume is depleted.

During resuscitation, children are particularly prone to:

- hypoglycaemia
- hyponatraemia, which may cause cerebral oedema.

These problems need to be anticipated.

Long-term effects

It is important to consider the sequelae of a major life-threatening and disfiguring injury on the body and psyche of a growing patient. The effect of growth on the effects of scars and contractures needs to be anticipated and treated early.

- Psychological upset is difficult to deal with and requires a great deal of support.
- Major burns cause growth delay that never fully recovers.

- Breast burns have the potential to recover well even if the nipple–areolar complex seems badly burnt. Acute burn management should be conservative to maximize survival of the breast bud by allowing the burn to demarcate before carrying out careful tangential debridement. However, subsequent contractures should be managed aggressively, with timely release and reconstruction with graft or flap repair to allow the greatest potential for normal development.

Toxic shock syndrome

Staphylococcus aureus colonizes burns wounds within 1–2 days. In very rare occasions, some strains produce toxic shock syndrome toxin (TSST-1, 75%) or staphylococcal enterotoxins (25%), which are absorbed. TSST-1 is described as a 'superantigen' as it overstimulates T lymphocytes, causing a wide range of effects. The burns involved are often small; children are said to be especially susceptible to the disease due to a lack of immunity.

- Prodrome: 24–48h of diarrhoea, vomiting, malaise and pyrexia
- Rash
- Raised leukocyte count, raised INR, low calcium and low albumin
- Shock (mortality of 50%).

Management involves:

- Aggressive resuscitation, invasive monitoring e.g. CVP is recommended
- Cleaning the infected wound
- Administration of antibiotics: clindamycin is first line for invasive group A streptococcal infections; penicillins are not particularly effective. Some recommend a combination with a beta-lactamase resistant anti-staphylococcal antibiotic.
- FFP/blood
- Specific antitoxin (commercial preparations—pooled immunoglobulin reserved for refractory cases).

The role of prevention with prophylactic antibiotics is controversial and is not common practice. It is more important to have a high index of suspicion and to advise parents of the warning signs prior to discharge.

Non-accidental injury (NAI)

There are certain features in a burn that should raise suspicions that a burn has been deliberately inflicted:

- history inconsistent with injury
- changing story
- delay in presentation
- previous injuries
- glove and stocking distribution
- scalds
- cigarette burns.

Further reading

Meyer WJ III, Blakeney P, Russell W et al. Psychological problems reported by young adults who were burned as children. *J Burn Care Rehabil* 2004; **25**:98–106.

Related topic of interest

• Acute burns.

Parotid gland tumours

The name 'parotid' comes from the Greek for 'near the ear'. Its most important relation is with the facial nerve; 80% of the gland lies superficial to it.

Lumps in the parotid gland are 80% likely to be benign, whereas with submandibular gland lumps, the incidence of benign lesions is 50% and in the sublingual glands, it is 20%, i.e. such lesions are more likely to be malignant. Parotid lumps are more likely to be malignant in children.

- 80% of salivary gland tumours are in the parotid
- 80% of parotid lumps are benign
- 80% of benign parotid tumours are pleiomorphic adenomas.

There are certain features in a parotid lump that suggest it may be malignant:

- invasion of the facial nerve giving rise to facial palsy or pain
- invasion of the parotid duct causing obstruction, infection or bleeding
- invasion of the muscles or the temporomandibular joint causing trismus.

Three-quarters of patients with these features have nodes at the time of presentation and on average survive less than 3 years.

The classification of parotid gland tumours is rather complex, e.g. WHO. The commonest benign and malignant lesions are discussed below.

Benign parotid tumours

Pleiomorphic salivary adenomas
Pleiomorphic salivary adenomas (PSAs) are sometimes called 'mixed tumours' due to the presence of epithelial and mesenchymal components in the tumour. These are the commonest benign parotid tumours and usually present as a slow-growing painless mass in the parotid, usually the tail of the glands, often noticed coincidentally while shaving or washing. Typical patients are 40–50 years old with a slight female predominance.

The standard treatment is a superficial parotidectomy. The tumour is surrounded by a delicate pseudocapsule formed by compressed normal glandular tissue with some tumour pseudopodia projecting into it. Simple enucleation is generally discouraged and will lead to recurrence rates of 25% or more, whereas excisional surgery taking a cuff of normal gland will reduce recurrence to 1–5%. Recurrence is more common if there was rupture of the tumour or if it was close to the facial nerve. The first chance is the best chance, as recurrences may be multifocal and re-operation has an increased risk to the facial nerve.

> The risk of malignant transformation to a carcinoma ex pleiomorphic adenoma (CXPA) is around 2–10% and presents as a sudden increase in size, pain, palsy and fixity, which generally occurs in a PSA after 10–15 years.

Adenolymphomas (Warthin's tumour)

Adenolymphomas are classically soft cystic lumps in the tail of the parotid in elderly (60–70 years) males (five times more commonly than in females), particularly in smokers, who have a 40× risk. It is more frequent in Orientals, for whom in some series it is more common than pleiomorphic adenomas (25–40%). It is bilateral/multifocal in 5–10% of patients. Recurrence is uncommon (2%) after treatment with a superficial parotidectomy. Some of the reported recurrences may be due to multifocal disease.

Malignant parotid tumours

Malignant parotid tumours occur mostly in the body of the parotid. They can either be primary or secondary (squamous cell carcinoma 40% and melanoma 45%, particularly from the scalp or ear).

Mucoepidermoid carcinomas

Mucoepidermoid carcinomas form one-third of malignant parotid tumours and 8% of all parotid tumours. The degree of histological differentiation influences its behaviour and prognosis.

- Well-differentiated carcinomas behave like pleiomorphic adenomas and rarely metastasize.
- Poorly differentiated tumours behave more like adenoid cystic carcinomas and are prone to local invasion and regional spread.

Treatment is usually aggressive excision followed by radiotherapy.

Adenoid cystic carcinomas

Adenoid cystic carcinomas make up one-fifth of malignant parotid tumours. There are a number of histological subtypes: cribose tumours have the best prognosis and solid tumours the worst, with tubular tumours being somewhere in between. Haematogenous spread to the lungs is more common than nodal spread. These tumours do not have a capsule. Aggressive excisional surgery and radiotherapy is the typical treatment; if the superficial parotidectomy specimen shows high-grade malignancy, a large tumour or nodal involvement, a completion total parotidectomy should be performed. However, there is a tendency for perineural invasion with skip lesions along the facial nerve and the observed propensity to recur, often after many years, raises some doubt whether a true 'cure' is possible. The clinical behaviour of the lesion is unpredictable; it is locally invasive but may be stable for many years.

Lymphomas

Parotid lymphomas occur in 5–10% of Warthin's tumours and often occur in patients with Sjögren's disease or hepatitis C infection. Chemotherapy is the treatment of choice rather than surgery.

Investigations

Imaging

MRI and CT provide nearly the same information with nearly 100% sensitivity, although most would agree that MRI (T2) is better than CT:

- for assessing tumour margins
- for distinguishing between benign and malignant disease
- not affected by amalgam artefact.

CT provides better detail of surrounding tissue including the duct. Imaging is especially useful in assessing recurrent disease that may be multifocal.

Fine needle aspiration cytology (FNAC)

The role of FNAC is controversial. In most cases, it provides little information that would change management. It may be useful in providing confirmatory results in:

- poor surgical candidates
- parotid lumps in patients with other malignancies or with lymphoma.

It is a very operator-dependent procedure—the best results are achieved with experienced cytopathologists. It is of little use in epithelial lesions for which the architecture is needed. Sensitivity can be rather low (75%), but specificity and overall accuracy is over 90%, therefore only positive results should be accepted. **Frozen sections** are at best 93% accurate, but depend greatly on the experience of the pathologist. They should not be totally relied upon; clinical impression is paramount.

Superficial parotidectomy

Superficial parotidectomy with facial nerve preservation can be viewed as a biopsy procedure for parotid lumps that will serve as adequate management in over 80%.

- Surgery is performed under a general anaesthetic and muscle relaxant is avoided; the use of nerve stimulators is common but not universal. It is certainly very useful to check the integrity of the nerve branches at the end of the operation. The common incision is a 'lazy S' or Blair incision along the preauricular crease down and looping behind the ear over the mastoid with a cervical incision two finger-breadths below the mandible in the direction of the hyoid.
- The skin flap is elevated from the parotid anteriorly.
- The parotid tail is separated from the muscles (sternomastoid and posterior belly of digastric). The great auricular nerve should be spared if possible. Injury to the posterior facial veins will lead to congestion of the gland and increased bleeding.
- The facial nerve is normally approached in an anterograde manner using the tragal pointer as a landmark—the facial nerve is 1 cm inferior and deep to it. There are alternative landmarks, such as the stylomastoid foramen and stylomastoid artery. The parotid is dissected away piecemeal from the nerve. Retrograde dissection may be needed in very large lesions that are difficult to retract; the distal branches are identified, e.g. the buccal branch above the parotid duct and the marginal mandibular over the facial vessels.

Surgery for malignant lesion is generally more extensive than for benign lesions and may require sacrifice of the facial nerve. The role of radiotherapy in benign disease is controversial, as the response rate is low and there is concern that it may cause malignant change. It may be useful for multifocally recurrent pleiomorphic adenomas and for malignant disease, especially adenoid cystic carcinoma.

Complications need to be carefully explained to patients:

- Frey's syndrome (gustatory sweating/auriculotemporal syndrome) is sweating over the parotid area when eating. It is due to severed secretomotor parasympathetic fibres connecting up with the auriculotemporal nerve, and may occur in 10–50% of cases, although some say that subclinical disease is almost universal. Treatment can be as simple as using antiperspirants or topical scopolamine. Surgery may be required in the form of dermofat grafts, fascial flaps (such as fascia lata or fascia temporalis) or neurectomy. A newer treatment is botulinum toxin injection.
- Facial nerve palsy is usually only temporary (5%) but is permanent in a small number (1%). The risk is increased with re-operation (15–40%).
- Parotid fistula.
- Haematomas/seromas and wound infection occur in around 2–6%.

Further reading

Que Hee CG, Perry CF. Fine-needle aspiration cytology of parotid tumours: is it useful? *Aust NZ J Surg* 2001; **71:**345–8.

Premalignant lesions

These are lesions that are benign but show cellular changes such as dysplasia or atypia that are not yet frankly malignant.

- If left untreated there is a recognized risk of progression to frankly invasive malignancy, although not all cases will become malignant (see Table 1).
- If adequately treated, overt cancer can be prevented.
- Cancers that arise from premalignant lesions may be more aggressive than de novo cancers.

Table 1 Common premalignant lesions.

Lesion	Cancer risk and comments
Actinic keratosis (solar keratosis)	• Rough scaly slightly red lesions in sun-exposed areas that show cellular dysplasia and atypia. These are fairly common in the elderly. • A large proportion will progress eventually to squamous cell carcinoma (SCC) in situ, with 20% becoming frankly invasive; these tend to be **less** aggressive with very little metastatic potential. • They can be treated with cryotherapy (probably the commonest modality overall), surgically or with topical 5-fluorouracil (5-FU).
Leukoplakia	• These are white patches of hyperkeratosis found commonly on the oral mucosa, but may also be found in the vulva. • The aetiology is unknown; most are idiopathic, but in some it may be related to recurrent irritation from sharp teeth, tobacco smoke, etc. Some may regress if the cause is removed. 10–20% will progress to SCC, particularly if there is ulceration, nodules or verrucous change. Tumours that arise from Leukoplakin tend to be more aggressive. • Biopsy is mandatory and excision is recommended. Toludine blue staining can be used as an adjunct to guide biopsy of the most dysplastic areas. • Relapses are common.
Erythroplakia	• These are flat, slightly raised red velvety lesions; the colour is due to the loss of orthokeratin. Lesions may be granular or mixed with leukoplakia. • There is greater malignant potential than leukoplakia; the risk is about 50%. • Early excision is recommended.
Bowens disease	• This is a disease of the elderly and presents with scaly plaques that can be found anywhere but are commonly found on the trunk, legs and arms. It may be mistaken for psoriasis.

Table 1 *continued.*

Lesion	Cancer risk and comments
	• This is squamous cell carcinoma in situ, i.e. no dermal invasion, and therefore strictly is not premalignant. 3–11% progress to frankly invasive SCC and such lesions tend to be more aggressive than usual with a tendency to metastasize early. • It is histologically indistinguishable from erythroplasia of Queyrat, which is seen on the glans, inner prepuce, vulva or oral mucosa.

Further reading

Lober BA, Fenske NA. Optimum treatment strategies for actinic keratosis (intraepidermal squamous cell carcinoma). *Am J Clin Dermatol* 2004; **5:**395–401.

Pressure sores

This condition is often called a decubitus ulcer from the Latin 'decumbere' meaning 'to lie down', but this is a misnomer as the commonest sores are ischial sores that occur in the seated (i.e. the wheelchair bound). For similar reasons, the term 'bed sore' is not applicable in all cases.

Pressure sores are most common in the elderly (70% are in the over-70s) and neurologically impaired; it accounts for 6% of deaths on geriatrics wards and 7–8% of the deaths in paraplegics. The commonest type is the ischial sore (30%), then the greater trochanteric and the sacral (20% each) and the heel 10%, with the remainder consisting of sores on the malleoli and occiput.

Causes

The most important causative factor is prolonged excessive **pressure**. When the extrinsic pressure exceeds the capillary pressure of 32 mmHg, vessels are occluded and blood flow to the tissue stops. In the 'normal' person, this ischaemia would cause pain and prompt a shift in position. In the 'compromised', this protective action may not be possible. Changes can be obviated if the pressure can be relieved for 5 min every 2 h, but if the pressure is persistent, then necrosis and ulceration will result.

Muscle is more susceptible to ischaemia than skin. Therefore, the skin injury seen is often just the tip of the iceberg; the loss of tissue is cone-shaped with the apex at the skin. Concomitant factors such as low-level bacterial infection increase the susceptibility of skin to pressure, and in turn pressure may also reduce resistance to infection.

Other contributing factors include:

Friction and shear—mechanical stress may cause angulation of vessels that occludes flow. Certain intrinsic features of the patient will also increase the risk of developing pressure sores:

- malnutrition—most important
- incontinence
- altered sensation and consciousness
- advanced age.

The importance of these risk factors is reflected in their inclusion in the numerous risk scales that are used, such as the Norton, Braden and Waterlow scales. It is important to realize that these scales only assess the general condition of the patient and their risk of developing bed sores; in the end, it is actually the standard of care that has the greatest contribution.

It is common to grade the sore by the extent of visible destruction.

Stage 1—non-blanching erythema (1 h after relief of pressure), epidermis is unbroken

Stage 2—partial-thickness skin loss, with a shallow ulcer or blister

Stage 3—full-thickness skin loss, up to the fascia

Stage 4—through the fascia, extensive deep destruction may involve muscle, bone and joints

Management

Prevention is important and infinitely preferable. Attention needs to be paid to the risk factors: simple turning at irregular intervals is effective. This aims to distribute the weight evenly. Clinitron beds are effective for supine patients, but are very bulky and may cause electrolyte and water loss and in addition, it may impair pulmonary toilet in those with breathing problems.

Treatment of pressure sores can be difficult and prolonged. It is important to investigate fully and to identify and correct any correctible predisposing factors, which will also be important in reducing recurrence:

- Optimize nutrition.
- Correct anaemia.
- Treat infection (commonly *Staphylococcus aureus*, proteus, pseudomonas, bacteroides) with oral antibiotics. Colonization is common and proof of actual infection requires a deep biopsy.
- Treat spasm (common in spinal cord injury) as sores will inevitably recur if the spasm is not relieved. Valium, baclofen and dantrolene may be useful in some; in others surgery may be required to relieve spasm and contractures.
- Osteomyelitis needs to be actively excluded.
- X-rays, bone scans or biopsies may be needed.

Stage 1 and 2: dressings with pressure management

The aim of dressings is to keep the wound moist, but at the same time to remove excess exudates. There is a wide range of dressings available and without properly controlled trials it is difficult to establish how much better one dressing is over another. Common regimes include alginates and foams, sequentially followed by hydrogels/hydrocolloids. Patient acceptance is affected by:

- leakage and odours that affect social interaction
- length of time between changes for convenience
- pain especially during changes.

Vacuum closure can be useful.

Stage 3 and 4: surgery

Surgery may not always be appropriate—it is not usually indicated in deteriorating or terminal patients. It is most useful for young patients who are motivated and clinically stable and where postoperative prevention of recurrence is possible. Incontinent patients may need faecal or urinary diversion to improve wound care.

Principles (after Conway):

- The wound must be clean prior to surgery (whirlpool baths), although this will make the wound appear bigger. The use of pulsatile lavage is undergoing evaluation in controlled trials.
- Formal debridement is needed to remove dead tissue, bursae and calcified tissue and to smooth down bony surfaces.
- Large flaps should be used, but always try to maintain future options; use flaps that can be re-advanced in cases of recurrence. Dead spaces should be filled in a tension-free manner.

- There is evidence that fasciocutaneous flaps are better, with less recurrence than myocutaneous flaps (muscle is more sensitive to ischaemia and will atrophy with time). Donor areas should be covered with a thick split-skin graft if they cannot be closed primarily.
- Suture lines should be placed away from direct pressure. Sutures can be left for 3 weeks or more.
- Large drains are kept in place for 2 weeks.
- Optimize nutrition and avoid pressure.

The postoperative period is prolonged but is an important part of the whole procedure. Traditionally, the patient was immobilized for up to 8 weeks, but prospective trials in 1997 have shown no difference between 2 or 3 weeks of immobility before gradual mobilization. Overall short-term surgical results are good, but sores may recur, especially in the elderly, the debilitated or those who have suffered trauma.

Sacral sores
These usually have just a small dead space and fasciocutaneous flaps are suitable.

- Gluteus maximus musculocutaneous flaps can be used as bilateral VY advancement based on the superior gluteal artery (but cannot be reused) or as a rotation flap. The insertion to the greater trochanter can be sacrificed to increase flap excursion in non-ambulatory patients.
- Transverse lumbosacral artery flap.

Ischial sores
Ischial sores have a larger dead space and are more likely to need muscle to provide bulk and are some of the most difficult to treat. Excessive excision of the ischial tuberosity is not beneficial and will lead to increased pressure on the contralateral side.

- first choice is often the gluteal thigh rotation fasciocutaneous flap based on the inferior gluteal artery
- VY flaps, e.g. semitendinosus based on the first profunda femoris perforator
- TFL
- Tensor fascia lata (TFL) is supplied by the terminal branch of the lateral circumflex femoral artery from profunda femoris.

Greater trochanter
- TFL
- vastus lateralis flap based on first descending branch of the lateral circumflex artery
- gluteal thigh flap.

Further reading

Isik FF, Engrav LH, Rand RP et al. Reducing the period of immobilization following pressure sore surgery: a prospective randomized trial. *Plast Reconstr Surg* 1997; **100**:350–4.

Related topic of interest

- Vacuum wound closure.

Prominent ears

Prominent ears can cause a great deal of distress to the patient due to the embarrassment and teasing that may be encountered. This is determined in a great part by the local culture and how it views the 'problem'; consequently, the rates of surgery vary greatly between different populations.

Management

The preoperative assessment is vital.

- It is important to establish the reasons for surgery. In adults this is fairly straightforward; however, with children, parental concerns are an additional factor. It is preferable to have a child old enough to understand and actually want the treatment; this ensures a greater level of cooperation. Psychological assessment may be necessary.
- The anatomical problem, which may have several different components needs to be established. The most common problems are:
  —flattened antihelix
  —excessively deep conchae
  —flat conchoscaphal angle
  —other problems include a prominent mastoid; the protrusion of the lower or upper pole may contribute to the overall appearance of prominence.
- An honest explanation of the surgery and its complications and limitations is mandatory. Preoperative photographs are advisable.

Non-surgical treatment

It is suggested that increased maternal oestrogen levels in the neonate keeps the cartilage malleable, and that as levels drop after 72 h, the cartilage becomes less malleable. There are reports that splintage within this early window may be effective (Matsuo et al. 1989), particularly for Stahl bars (Aki et al. 2000), although the results are not wholly conclusive. There are practical issues as the splintage system needs to be used over several months, taking particular care with pressure points.

Surgery

There are many different surgical techniques (called pinnaplasty or otoplasty) that consist of different combinations of:

- cartilage moulding
- suturing
- excision.

The surgery can be performed under a local anaesthetic for adults and mature, motivated children. Many surgeons prefer to use general anaesthesia.

Cartilage moulding—the Gibson principle states that cartilage scored or abraded on one surface will bend away from that surface. This may be performed in an 'open' or 'closed' (actually via small incisions) manner and is an integral part of many techniques.

Suturing

- **Conchal-fossa**—these are the Mustarde sutures that aim to create an antihelical fold. Clear monofilament sutures on cutting or taper-cutting needles are used to place mattress sutures that are just tight enough to create the fold—the aim is not to coapt the cartilage surfaces of the concha and scaphoid fossa. They are usually placed from behind (medial surface) but can be placed anteriorly via very small incisions.
- **Concha-mastoid**—this aims to reduce the projection of a deep concha. After dissection of connective tissue, muscles and ligaments from the postauricular area, mattress sutures are placed between the conchal cartilage and the mastoid process. The sutures need to be stronger than those used for the Mustarde stitch.

Excision

- Posterior skin—resection of a portion of the postauricular skin is part of many techniques. A common incision pattern is the dumbbell shape; it is primarily for access, though it removes redundant skin. An operation that relies on skin excision alone will almost inevitably lead to recurrence.
- Excision of conchal cartilage can be performed if the concha is excessively deep.

Postoperative care

- Soft dressings, e.g. acraflavin wool, are moulded to conform to the newly created contours. Some evidence suggests that conchal dressings contribute to postoperative nausea.
- A head bandage is often used but is not deemed to be absolutely necessary.
- Check for bleeding or shift in dressings; some routinely replace dressings on the first postoperative day; other surgeons only replace them as necessary.
- Headbands or other support is used for variable lengths of time (weeks to months) but is particularly important in children.

Complications

- Haematoma (1%). Sudden increase in pain postoperatively suggests a haematoma and inspection of the ear is mandatory. Failing to adequately treat a haematoma will lead to cartilage necrosis. Adrenaline (epinephrine) infiltration can be safely used without any increase in the complication rate.
- Infection is rare. The operation is 'clean' but prophylactic antibiotics are commonly given due to the potentially serious sequelae of chondritis.
- Scarring problems may arise and are less common in Caucasians (2%) compared to Afro-Caribbeans (11%).

- Recurrence and under- or overcorrection of the abnormality is a possibility (4%) that the patient must be made aware of. Symmetry cannot be guaranteed.
- Small irregularities, if detected early, may be corrected by moulding. Abnormalities such as the 'hidden helix' (due to overcorrection) and 'telephone deformity' may result.

Further reading

Aki FE, Kaimoto CL, Katayama ML et al. Correction of Stahl's Ear. *Aesthetic Plastic Surgery* 2000; **24(5):**382–5.

Kelley P, Hollier L, Stal S. Otoplasty: evaluation, technique, and review. *J Craniofac Surg* 2003; **14:**643–53.

Matsuo K, Hirose T. A splint for non surgical correction of cryptotia. *Eur J Plast Surg* 1989; **12:**187–8.

Rhinoplasty

The aim of rhinoplasty is to achieve a natural looking nose that blends in with the rest of the face. The nose should be consistent with the patient's ethnic identity.

Patients seeking surgery include those with structural abnormality causing nasal dysfunction or deformity, and those with cosmetic concerns.

- Functional
- Cosmetic:
  —objective (obvious deformity or asymmetry)
  —subjective (more subtle, nose does not fit with rest of the face).

History

It is vital to fully assess the patient's wishes to see if their expectations are realistic.
- Previous trauma/surgery
- Evidence of nasal disease, e.g. epistaxis, rhinitis, nasal obstruction or anosmia
- Use of nasal drugs, both prescribed and 'recreational', e.g. cocaine.

Examination

A systematic assessment of the skeleton (bone and cartilage) and the soft tissue envelope is needed.

- **Overall shape of the nose**, comparing it to skeletal proportions of the face, including the dentition and forehead. A lateral view with smiling tends to accentuate 'problems'
  —dorsum: height, width and humps
  —**angles**: septal, nasofrontal, tip-collumella, nasolabial (90–95° males, 100–105° females)
  —**tip**: nasal tip projection (from nasal spine to tip), nasal length (from root just below eyelash line to tip and occupies central third of the face) and tip definition.
- **Skin quality**—thicker nasal skin can conceal underlying structures, e.g. alloplastic implants
- **Septal deviation and quality** of cartilage for graft availability; size of inferior turbinate
- **Internal valve**—this is the area between the septum and the caudal border of the upper lateral cartilage and it must be protected to preserve the flexibility and patency of the valve. Intranasal examination includes assessment of nasal obstruction; potential collapse of the internal valve can be assessed with lateral traction (Cottle manoeuvre).

Preoperative photographs are important.

There are ethnic/racial differences in the nasal shape: in general, there is a lack of skeletal support in non-Caucasians that produces a broad flat nose, wider-based alae with flared and horizontal nostrils, and less tip projection.

Surgery

Rhinoplasty can be performed under either local anaesthesia and sedation or general anaesthesia. Intraoperative bleeding is reduced by vasoconstriction with adrenaline (epinephrine) injection (using only small amounts to avoid distortion), xylometazoline or cocaine paste.

Surgical techniques
- **Closed**—this is the most frequently used approach and is regarded as the 'traditional' approach. It is adequate for most patients.
- **Open**—transverse columellar and marginal incisions with degloving gives good exposure and so is especially useful for extensive nasal tip work. Accurate cartilage visualization, especially where the cartilages are distorted, e.g. in a cleft nose, is important to place grafts precisely and for rhinoplasty in non-Caucasians that may be more challenging. Although operative time is longer, the open technique may be better for the inexperienced and also for teaching. However, it involves extra dissection that is probably unnecessary if no nasal tip work is needed; the resultant tip oedema can last for months.

Dorsum
Reduction: a prominent dorsal hump is a common problem.

- Smooth down humps with a rasp, osteotome or saw; the rasp is easier to use for beginners.
- A broad bridge can be narrowed: the sides are in-fractured after weakening the base with osteotomes (transnasal or transcutaneous) or a saw.
- Augmentation is more commonly needed in South East Asians (e.g. Southern Chinese, Malays); Caucasians tend to need reductions.

Augmentation: there are different methods of augmenting the dorsum.
Injections of paraffin or liquid silicone are rarely performed now except by non-surgeons. Prior infection is a contraindication to augmentation as the infection rate nears 40%.

Implants

- **Alloplastic**—silicone, proplast, teflon. The procedure is quicker, with no donor site morbidity, but can be complicated by extrusion and infection. In addition, the implant may be palpable or visible and an inflammatory reaction can lead to bad scarring in a minority. Medpor (porous high-density polyethylene [PHDPE]) is said to be more rigid, providing more support, and also encourages vascular ingrowth, which may be beneficial; but information on long-term results is lacking.
- **Autogenous**—cartilage (septum, ear, rib, etc.) or bone (calvarium, iliac, etc.). In Caucasians, autogenous cartilage is usually used in preference to bone, with alloplastic materials being a less frequent option. However, in Asians, silastic implants are the commonest material used, partly because patients have little autogenous tissue and also because they tend to tolerate implants better due in part to the thicker skin.

Nasal tip

The tip may be refined in many different ways, but most involve:

1. suture techniques, especially involving alar cartilage of the medial crura
2. cartilage grafts: onlay, umbrella graft (with a strut into columella) and spreader grafts.

Postoperative care

- Nasal packing is a common practice, but may not be necessary; it does not need to be inserted very deeply into the nose. Packing is generally kept for 1–3 days, and prophylactic antibiotics should be given concomitantly. External splints, if used, can be removed after a week.
- Antibiotics coverage is required if an implant has been used.

Bruising and nasal blockage for up to 2 weeks are to be expected. Swelling may be prolonged.

Complications

Complications occur in 4–20% of patients.

- Asymmetry, irregularity, e.g. 'open roof', 'rocker' or 'step' deformity
- Postoperative deformity requiring secondary surgery occurs in 5–10%
- Under- or overcorrection
- Haemorrhage in 4% is usually minor.

- Numb upper alveolus
- Nasal obstruction
- Septal perforation.

For those patients with implants:

- Infection can occur many months after surgery. It may be possible to eradicate the infection with broad-spectrum antibiotics and irrigation; but many eventually need removal of the implant. Further surgery is generally delayed for 6–9 months.
- Migration can occur.
- If an implant is extruding, then sterility has been compromised and it should be removed.

Further reading

Adamson PA, Galli SK. Rhinoplasty approaches: current state of the art. *Arch Facial Plast Surg* 2005; **7**:32–7.

Skin grafts

A skin graft is a piece of skin taken from one part of the body, detached from its blood supply, and then transferred to another part of the body that allows its re-incorporation. This is an autograft.

- Allograft—transplant from an individual of the same species with a different genotype
- Xenograft—transplant from an individual of a different species.

Early adhesion of the graft is due to fibrin, but with no inherent blood supply, the graft will die unless nutrition to the cells is re-established. The process of a graft being accepted at the recipient site is called 'take'. The details have not been fully elucidated, although a series of steps have been suggested.

- **Imbibition** (24–48h)—during this stage, the graft relies on nutrients reaching it by passive means; the graft 'drinks' from the recipient bed. The graft increases in weight and volume during this stage.
- **Inosculation**—some vascularity is re-established by blood vessels in the recipient bed connecting to vessels in the graft dermis. This has been demonstrated in experiments with Indian ink, although it is not clear how this occurs. The graft begins to look pink at this stage.
- **Revascularization**—after 4–7 days, new vessels form due to host endothelium ingrowth into the graft.

The relative contributions of inosculation and revascularization are unclear.

It follows that the recipient bed needs to be sufficiently vascular to support a graft. Relatively avascular structures such as bare bone/tendon/cartilage and to a lesser extent, nerves, will not support grafts reliably.

In the presence of an adequately vascular bed, the commonest reasons for skin graft failure are:

- **Haematoma/seroma**—the fluid raises the graft away from the vascular bed, limiting the transfer of nutrients. This can be reduced by careful haemostasis (the dermal component of the graft is haemostatic, but this will not stop more profuse bleeding). Making fenestrations in the graft either by hand or by machine meshing will allow drainage of potential collections but will leave unattractive marks. A pressure dressing or a tie-over dressing may also help; small collections may be carefully 'rolled out'. Inspecting a graft early i.e. before the 4th day may catch these problems early.
- **Shearing**—shearing will disrupt vascular connections. This problem is reduced by immobilizing the graft: securing the periphery with sutures, glue or staples, and fixing the graft to the bed (quilting sutures). A 'tie over' dressing may be used and a splint reduces movement near joints. A suction dressing may be used for grafts in difficult areas such as the perineum. With a cooperative patient, an exposed graft may be an option and has the benefits of being able to inspect the graft continuously.
- **Infection**—a clean bed is needed; small amounts of colonization of most bacteria are generally not important, but heavy growth of bacteria (10^5 organisms per gram

of tissue), or moderate growth of streptococcus with its lysins will lead to graft failure. There is a case for swabbing the wounds prior to elective surgery and administering prophylactic antibiotics.

Total failure is usually due to the graft being placed upside down on the recipient bed; the waterproof stratum corneum will not allow nutrients to pass to reach the graft cells.

Thickness of grafts

Skin grafts consist of the epidermis and a variable amount of dermis. Depending on the amount of dermis taken, skin grafts can be classified as:

- **Partial-thickness grafts**, usually called **split skin grafts** (SSGs, Thiersch graft), are where only part of the dermis is taken, along with the epidermis. The donor site will usually heal spontaneously, since the epidermal regenerative capacity resides in the dermal appendages (the sebaceous glands, sweat glands and hair follicles) left behind. The graft can be taken by hand with a Watson skin graft knife or by a powered dermatome. The thickness of the graft can be assessed by the translucency of the graft and the bleeding pattern from the donor—fine punctuate bleeding suggests a thin graft has been taken. Some markings or scarring may be left at the donor depending on the depth of graft taken. The thicker the split-thickness graft, the slower it will take, resembling a full-thickness graft.
- **Full-thickness grafts** (Wolfe graft, FTSGs) have all the dermis with all its appendages. It is usually taken by hand with a blade and often requires defatting. The donor will not heal, and consequently requires primary closure or possibly a SSG.

Full-thickness skin grafts are 'superior' to SSGs because they have the full thickness of the skin.

- The appearance is better. In addition, the donor can be closed to a linear scar.
- The graft is more durable and functionality is more likely to be preserved:
  —SSGs are typically very dry and may require emollients. FTSGs are less dry as the sweat glands are maintained, and when re-innervated, their function approaches that of the recipient.
  —Re-innervation leads to sensory return that begins after around 4 weeks, with pain recovering before light touch or temperature.
- There is less contraction:
  —Primary contraction is the immediate recoil or shrinkage of a graft once taken and is due to elastin in the dermis.
  —Secondary contraction is late contraction after the skin graft has taken and healed; it is related to myofibroblast activity that is said to be inhibited by dermal components.
  —Therefore, SSGs will have less primary contraction (10% vs 40%) but more secondary contraction than FTSGs, but overall, SSGs contract more than FTSGs.

However, the amount of available FTSG is limited, whereas a SSG donor area will heal and the harvesting of more skin may be possible, depending on the thickness of dermis left behind.

Meshing

Skin grafts can be meshed to:

- expand the area of coverage
- improve contouring and allow drainage of exudates.

Multiple holes in the graft are made by a machine that allows the skin to open up with lateral traction like a net. The ratio of expansion can be varied. With a wider mesh (>3–4× expansion), the interstices will heal more slowly by re-epithelialization from the sides, and desiccation of the central part makes scarring more likely. In order to reduce desiccation and promote healing, the meshed skin can be covered by a layer of allograft (the sandwich graft technique), or with cultured keratinocytes.

Excess skin graft may be stored in a fridge at 4°C for up to a week (or kept in specific medium for several weeks, or in liquid nitrogen for much longer, but these latter options are impractical).

Composite grafts

A composite graft is a graft that contains a combination of tissues such as skin, fat, and sometimes the underlying cartilage from the donor site. It is used when extra support is needed, e.g. using auricular skin and cartilage to replace nasal defects. It doesn't have its own blood supply and due to the thickness of the tissues that must be nourished by passive means initially, survival is less predictable than for simple skin grafts—the upper limit is usually regarded as 1–1.5 cm. The survival of the cartilage component may be improved by adding a large skin island. There is some evidence that postoperative cooling may actually enhance healing, contrary to the conventional practice of keeping them warm. The data on hyperbaric oxygen are inconclusive.

Further reading

Adams C, Ratner D. Composite and free cartilage grafting. *Dermatol Clin* 2005; **23:**129–40.

Related topic of interest

- Vacuum wound closure.

Squamous cell carcinomas

The incidence of squamous cell carcinomas (SCCs) is four times less than basal cell carcinoma (BCC) in Caucasians. SCCs typically occur on the sun-exposed skin of late middle-aged or elderly males (2:1). The incidence increases for every 10° of latitude closer to the equator.

The appearance can be quite variable depending in part on the degree of differentiation.

- Scaly red patches resembling Bowens
- Classic keratotic papule, with or without a keratin horn or ulceration
- Nodular.

Keratin pearls are a characteristic histological finding in the more-differentiated SCCs.

Risk factors

- **Ultraviolet light B** (UVB) in sunlight—thymidine dimers are formed causing point mutations; p53 mutations have been reported as well. The interaction between complexion/skin type and cumulative sun exposure, especially that causing sunburns, is important. PUVA (psoralen and ultraviolet A) treatment for psoriasis is also a risk factor.
- Irradiation was used in the past to treat a variety of benign conditions, including acne and ringworm, before its risks were known. It continues to be part of the treatment of many malignancies; in thyroid cancer and lymphoma in particular, the patients are typically younger.
- Chronic wounds. Osteomyelitis sinus, burns scar, ulcers, etc.—Marjolin's ulcer. A high degree of suspicion is required to be aware of any change in the lesion. The prognosis is worse as the diagnosis is often delayed and these tumours are generally more aggressive.
- Premalignant conditions may lead to SCCs—actinic keratosis, Bowen's disease and leukoplakia.
- Immunosuppression—a third of transplant patients develop SCCs; that are often multiple.
- Xeroderma pigmentosa (XP) and albinism.

Keratoacanthoma (KA) is an important differential diagnosis. These are fast-growing nodular lesions that classically involute within months but sometimes with significant scarring. It is regarded by some as a well-differentiated subset of SCC, and is sometimes referred to as SCC, keratoacanthoma type. Histologically, there will be similarities to SCC, but it will show signs of involution. It is generally NOT appropriate to wait and see if a potential keratoacanthoma will involute and early surgical excision is preferable.

Management

It is important to realize that SCCs are potentially serious problems with significant chances of nodal and distant metastasis and mortality, particularly if recurrent. The first chance is the best chance, so it is important to aim for complete resection. Continued follow-up is important to detect recurrences and new tumours that may occur due to the field effect.

- History and examination is important, as always.
- Check for lymphadenopathy and distant metastasis. The risk of occult lymph nodes in SCCs is 2–3% overall and about 5% of SCCs will metastasize. Prognosis is closely related to the TNM stage.

Tumours with certain features are said to be 'high risk' with increased risk of recurrence and metastasis; in these tumours, the rate of metastasis is nearly 30% and the mortality rate is 30%.

- SCCs that arise due to risk factors other than ultraviolet light, including immunosuppression, XP and Marjolin's
- big lesions (>2 cm), thick lesions (the depth of invasion is actually a good prognostic indicator), less well differentiated (risk of recurrence in well-differentiated lesions is 7% compared to 28% in the poorly differentiated) and evidence of perineural and vascular invasion.

Treatment

For selected early lesions, options include:

- cryotherapy for the elderly or for in situ disease/actinic keratosis
- curettage and electrodesiccation
- radiation is not recommended as a primary treatment modality, but has a role as an adjunctive treatment.

In the majority of patients, surgery is the mainstay of treatment. Commonly, margins of 5 mm are taken on the face and 1 cm elsewhere, but there is little hard evidence to support this. Zitelli suggests 4 mm for low-risk lesions and 6 mm for high-risk lesions. Complete margin control, i.e. Moh's micrographic surgery, is useful for high-risk tumours and recurrences.

Further reading

Cohen EE. Novel therapeutic targets in squamous cell carcinoma of the head and neck. *Semin Oncol* 2004; **31:**755–68.

Related topics of interest

- Basal cell carcinoma
- Melanoma
- Premalignant lesions
- Ultraviolet light.

Stevens–Johnson syndrome

There is some disagreement about the relationship of Stevens–Johnson syndrome (SJS) to erythema multiforme (EM). Some regard SJS as a severe form of EM (i.e. EM majus), but it has become apparent recently that despite the similarities, there are notable differences between SJS and EM (see Table 1). Older literature that does not make this distinction needs to be interpreted carefully.

Toxic epidermal necrolysis (TEN) is a severe variant of SJS in which the extent of blistering is more than 30% of the body surface area, whereas in SJS it is less than 10%. TEN is consequently associated with a greater mortality (up to 40%) and with a greater risk of sepsis, renal failure, gastrointestinal bleeding and pneumonia. Some cases show overlap of features. Overall mortality is 3–15%.

The underlying problem in SJS/TEN seems to be related to immunity; some describe it as an immune-complex disorder with type IV (delayed) hypersensitivity; an association with autoimmune disorders such as lupus and HLA linkage has been suggested.

The condition is often preceded by a non-specific upper respiratory tract infection, with a prodrome of fever, dullness and malaise. See Table 2 for the clinical features of SJS/TEN.

Causes

- **Drugs**—SJS can be caused by almost any drug, but penicillins, phenytoin and sulfa/sulfonamide drugs are responsible for nearly two-thirds of these cases. Symptoms can appear up to 8 weeks after starting the suspected medication.

Table 1 Differences between erythema multiforme and SJS/TEN.

Erythema multiforme	SJS/TEN
Typically target lesions on extensor surfaces and dorsum of hands. Often symmetrical in distribution	Larger lesions with more blistering. Subcutaneous oedema is rare, unlike burns
Younger males more frequently affected 3:2	Female predominance
Frequent relapse	Relapse less common
Less fever	Fever is more frequently seen
Less mucosal involvement in general	Almost all have mucosal involvement
Associated with infections (mycoplasma)	Drugs are a common cause; risk increases with age and may be related to the polypharmacy in this group. Often idiosyncratic, occurrence is less predictable

Table 2 Clinical features of SJS/TEN.

Affected area	Features
Skin	Skin lesions appear abruptly, starting as a non-pruritic flat/macular rash that develops central blisters or necrosis. Individual lesions heal within 1–2 weeks, but new lesions can appear in crops for 2–3 weeks. More extensive blistering and desquamation leaves open wounds that are vulnerable to infection (which may present as a high fever or a worsening wound). Infected wounds have an increased risk of scar complications. **Nikolski sign**: skin lesions wrinkle or separate with slight lateral pressure. As only the epidermis sloughs off healing is usually rapid
Eye (50%)	Anterior uveitis, ectropion and corneal ulceration that may lead to blindness in 5–10%, ectropion
Gastrointestinal	Oesophageal strictures
Genitourinary	Dysuria, vaginal stenosis
Respiratory	Bronchopneumonia, respiratory failure
Nasal	Crusting

- **Infections**—Approximately one-third of patients with SJS have an associated infection, commonly viral (herpes simplex mycoplasma and coxsackie) or bacterial (group A beta haemolytic streptococcus). HIV infection significantly increases the risk of developing SJS/TEN.
- **Malignancy.**

Drugs and malignancy are more common causes in adults/the elderly, and infections more common in children. About one-quarter of cases will have no obvious cause and will be labelled idiopathic.

The diagnosis can be made from the clinical features in most cases; definitive diagnosis can be provided by a skin biopsy demonstrating:

- epidermal necrosis with separation from the dermis
- subepidermal bullae
- perivascular lymphocyte infiltration.

Treatment is generally supportive and symptomatic. **There is no proven specific therapy.**

- Stop the suspected drug and avoid other unnecessary drugs.
- It is important to prevent and treat infection; manage wounds like burns using simple dressings with minimal trauma and mouthwash, etc. However, silver sulphadiazine should be avoided as it may precipitate the problem. Prophylactic antibiotics have not been shown to be useful.
- Fluid replacement is administered as dictated by the surface area involved and the patient's vital signs.

Some advocate systemic steroids, but this is not universally accepted. It may be useful if given early (24–48 h), but there is an increased risk of complications, e.g. from immunosuppression, increased risk of infection and gastrointestinal bleeding; it may mask sepsis and reduce healing. There are no randomized clinical trials of the effectiveness of steroids; their use is probably detrimental in late cases.

Other treatments have been used in small series of patients:

- Some have used plasmapheresis to remove the drug quicker, but there is little evidence to support its wider use.
- Cyclophosphamide and cyclosporin A need more evaluation.
- TNF-alpha overexpression has been noted, and this provided the rationale for thalidomide treatment, but its use seems to be associated with increased mortality.
- Immunoglobulins showed promise in early reports, but these have not been reproducible; furthermore, it is an expensive treatment and there is the risk of renal failure and aseptic meningitis.

Further reading

Schulz JT, Sheridan RL, Ryan CM et al. A 10-year experience with toxic epidermal necrolysis. *J Burn Care Rehabil* 2002; **21:**199–204.

Suturing

Principles of good suturing

Placing an incision within or parallel to a **relaxed skin tension line** (RSTL) will produce a better scar with less tendency to hypertrophic scarring than one that crosses these lines. RSTLs tend to lie perpendicular to the direction of pull of the underlying muscles. On the face, they are sometimes called wrinkle lines and can be made more obvious by asking the patient to contract their muscles. When incision lines running parallel to RSTLs cannot be made, then they should be curved/wavy or a series of z-plasties.

Excision/incision
- Incisions are made perpendicular to the plane of the skin to avoid shelving.
- An adequate length of ellipse is needed to avoid dog-ear formation; the length should be 2–4 times the width and the orientation should be parallel to an RSTL.

Suturing
- **Respect the tissues**—forceps may be toothed or non-toothed and skin hooks are the most atraumatic, but whichever method is used, one must always handle the skin carefully—avoid crushing the skin.
- **Everting the skin edges** allows maximal dermal apposition. Everted edges will flatten gradually, whereas inverted edges tend to remain inverted and look unattractive. To promote skin eversion, simple interrupted stitches should be placed so that the needle enters and exits the skin perpendicularly. Equal depth of tissue should be taken on either side to ensure a level wound.
- **Avoid tension in the wound**—dermal sutures provide most of the strength in wound closure, limiting scar stretching after skin sutures are removed. Skin sutures should not be tied too tightly; simple apposition of the edges is sufficient as postoperative oedema will increase tension and ischaemia may result.
- **Minimize infection risk** and wound ischaemia by using the minimum number of interrupted sutures or a subcuticular suture—as a general rule, the distance between simple interrupted stitches should equal their length.

Types of stitching
- Simple interrupted stitches are simple and precise.
- Mattress sutures (vertical or horizontal) are good for eversion, particularly where the skin is thin and unsupported, but can cause more ischaemia.
- Subcuticular sutures do not strangle the skin and do not leave stitch marks. Sutures can be left for longer periods to support the wound but it can be more difficult to be as precise as simple interrupted sutures.

Classification of suture material

- **Material**—synthetic vs natural.
- **Degradability**—absorbable vs non-absorbable. Absorbable sutures do not need to be removed but can cause more inflammation and tissue reaction. Most modern sutures are degraded by hydrolysis, whereas catgut is degraded by proteolysis.
- **Number of filaments**—monofilament vs braided. Braided sutures handle better but exhibit tissue drag that may cause damage. They have an increased risk of infection due to bacteria colonizing the crevices between filaments. Monofilaments are prone to 'memory' and knots are prone to unravelling and benefit from an extra throw.

Suture material

- Catgut is being used less and less due to its unreliable absorption time, and being an animal product (bovine intestine), it has a theoretical risk of transmitting infection. It has most use as a mucosal suture and chromatization can delay absorption more consistently. It is no longer supplied in the UK.
- Vicryl (polyglactin 910) is a synthetic absorbable braided suture that keeps its strength for 4 weeks and is used frequently as a dermal/intradermal suture but can 'spit' out.
- Monocryl (poliglecaprone) and PDS are both synthetic absorbable monofilament sutures; PDS keeps its strength for longer (months rather than weeks), which increases its tendency to spit out.
- Prolene is a synthetic non-absorbable monofilament and is used frequently for skin sutures, especially for 'subcuticular' sutures—it shows little tissue reaction and is easy to remove (it is smoother than nylon).

The numbering of sutures refers to their size—originally there were sizes 0–3, but with advances in production, thinner sutures had to be denoted with an extra '0', e.g. 6/0 which is finer than 3/0.

Needles

Needles are already swaged to reduce their profile and thus reduce tissue trauma. Needles may be described by their:

- curvature—straight, curved or J shaped
- profile—round bodied (for blood vessels and intestines, less tearing to reduce leakage), cutting (able to penetrate tough tissue such as skin), reverse cutting and taper cut. Blunt needles are sometimes used for fascia to reduce needle-stick injuries.

Removing sutures

A skin wound is waterproof after 48 hours. Skin sutures need to be removed at the correct time to prevent stitch marks due to epithelium spreading along beside the suture, forming a sinus tract; cross-hatching occurs due to prolonged tension on the skin. Appropriate timing of stitch removal and avoiding tension is more important than the choice of suture. General recommendations are:

- face and neck 5 days or less (3–4 days for the eyelids)
- scalp 10 days (if necessary, sutures may be left longer as the stitch marks will be covered by hair)

- arm 10 days
- legs 10–14 days
- back 10–14 days.

These times can be modified by factors such as anticipated delayed patient healing due to diabetes, etc.

To remove the suture, one end is cut flush with the skin (to avoid pulling through a significant length of exposed stitch material that will have been colonized by bacteria) and is pulled toward the incision line to reduce any tendency to 're-open' the wound. Some support in the form of steristrips or micropore may be advisable as the wound only has 5% of its original strength at 1 week; however, indefinite support is not effective as stretching of scars is mostly unpredictable.

Alternatives to excision

- Cryotherapy—liquid nitrogen is applied as a spray or with a cotton Q-tip for approximately 30s. Can be used for benign lesions as well as selected BCCs (prior tissue diagnosis is preferable). Scarring will still occur and hypopigmentation is a common sequela.
- Electrodesiccation and curettage: seem to be as effective as excision for removing selected lesions, including early BCCs. Electrodesiccation seems to add little to the 'curative' aspect, while causing most of the tissue damage.

Alternatives to sutures

It is important to note that the final result is determined by basic surgical principles, i.e. good quality wound edges, clean debrided wound and good apposition without tension, rather than the material per se.

- **Staples** allow rapid wound closure. In addition, there is minimal inflammatory reaction. However, it can be expensive.
- **Glue**—cyanoacrylates (Histacryl and Dermabond) are biodegradable adhesives that polymerize on contact—there is roughly 1 min available for fine adjustment of the edges. It should not be allowed to get inside the wound as it is cytotoxic. Glue is particularly useful for simple lacerations in children.
- **Steristrips**—they are easy to apply but are not as strong as sutures and will fall off when wet. It is important to avoid placing them under tension, particularly in the elderly with thin skin; traction dermatitis and even blistering can result.

Further reading

Lo S, Aslam N. A review of tissue glue use in facial lacerations: potential problems with wound selection in accident and emergency. *Eur J Emerg Med* 2004; **11:**277–9.

Related topics of interest

- Facial lacerations
- Local anaesthetics.

Tattoo removal

There are many reasons why people have their skin tattooed; a significant number will subsequently request removal when personal attitudes and circumstances change. Tattoos are usually classified as:

- **Professional tattoos**—there is uniform placement of pigment into the dermis. Modern tattoos can be bright/fluorescent, metallic or multicoloured.
- **Amateur tattoos**—less consistent in depth, but generally they are easier to remove because there is less ink and they are usually blue/black in colour.

The exact location of the tattoo dye has not been established with certainty; most studies suggest that it is inside fibroblasts, wrapped in a thin membrane and that permanence of colour may be due to the failure of the phagocytes to degrade the particles and also due to trapping of fibroblasts by fibrosis. A few studies suggest that some of the ink particles are extracellular. Clearing of the tattoo by most methods occurs by a mixture of pigment removal and being obscured by fibrosis.

Treatment options

Superficial destruction
A variety of mechanisms (mechanical, chemical and thermal) can be used to remove the superficial layers of skin. This removes some of the tattoo pigment and is often combined with the use of chemicals, e.g. tannic acid, oxalic acid or urea paste, to leech out more pigment from the denuded skin during the exudative phase. Such agents cause low-level inflammation that may promote phagocytic activity. These superficial methods are prone to leave residual pigmentation and will still produce scarring.

- Salabrasion—using salt is one of the oldest methods of tattoo removal.
- Dermabrasion—this can be quite bloody.
- Dermaplaning—the shaving of partial-thickness skin layers.
- Thermal infrared coagulator—this is supposedly specific for vessels (and so is promoted for use in vascular lesions as well as tattoos) but the results are similar to other non-specific methods, i.e. scarring and incomplete response.

Deep destruction
For those who can accept the scarring, quick one-stage procedures are available:

- Full-thickness excision and reconstruction with a variety of means, most commonly skin grafts.
- Ablative lasers such as CO_2 and argon target water in the tissues and so produce non-specific vaporization of surface layers. Scarring results from conductive heat damage of the deeper layers.

Q-switched (QS) lasers
Although initial experience with continuous wave lasers was promising, it was subsequently found to cause scarring as well as showing incomplete responses. A significant advance was the development of lasers capable of delivering nanosecond pulses that

cause photomechanical fragmentation of the pigment particles to a size that is more easily phagocytosed and degraded.

- One problem is splatter due to the force of the shockwave, and the debris may contain cells, viable viruses and other micro-organisms with infectivity.
- Several treatments (6–8 weeks apart) may be needed.

The wavelength of the laser light needs to be matched to the tattoo pigment, so several lasers are often needed to deal with multicoloured tattoos effectively (see Table 1). However, the exact composition of the ink is often unknown, contributing to the variable and inconsistent responses seen; on average, 50% of patients have a 50% response after 10 treatments.

Table 1   Suitable lasers for coloured tattoos.

Target colour	Effective lasers
Green	QS ruby, QS alexandrite
Red	QS frequency-doubled Nd-YAG
Black, blue–black	All tattoo lasers seem to be effective, particularly Nd-YAG

There are three major types of QS lasers used in tattoo removal (see Table 2):

- ruby (QSRL) 694 nm
- neodymium–yttrium–aluminium–garnet (Nd-YAG) 1064, which may be frequency doubled to 532 nm
- alexandrite 755 nm.

Table 2   Range of colours handled by different lasers.

Laser	Suitable for	Not suitable for
QS ruby	Green (blue)	Red
QS Nd-YAG	Black (dark blue)	Green
QS Nd-YAG frequency doubled	Red (black, dark blue, purple)	
QS alexandrite	Green (black, blue)	Orange/yellow

The longer wavelength of the Nd-YAG laser allows deeper penetration, and avoiding superficial structures makes it especially useful in darker skin, but at the expense of more splatter and bleeding. It works very well for black pigment, but effectiveness with other colours is limited compared to other lasers.

Complications of QS lasers

- Scarring is much less frequent than with other methods but is still possible.
- Incomplete response, particularly if the tattoo has a lot of green colour.

- Hypopigmentation (in around 50%) is usually temporary, but in a small number it may be permanent (especially with ruby lasers). Hyperpigmentation is less common and is related to the skin colour of the patient.
- Allergies are rare but may cause serious problems.
- Darkening may occur, especially with red or flesh-tone colours. Tattoos that have iron oxide or titanium oxide are prone to darkening; darkening in the former may be due to conversion to ferric oxide. Trials on a test patch are advisable.

Further reading

England RW, Vogel P, Hagan L. Immediate cutaneous hypersensitivity after treatment of tattoos with Nd-YAG laser: a case report and review of the literature. *Ann Allergy Asthma Immunol* 2002; **89:**215–17.

Related topics of interest

- Hair removal
- Lasers: principles.

Tissue expansion

New skin is generated when skin is subjected to prolonged stretching; this phenomenon is clearly seen during pregnancy. Similar results can be achieved by surgically implanting silastic expanders under the skin and then gradually expanding them by injecting with saline. Although most layers are thinned and hair density decreases, the epidermis is thickened. Two-thirds of the increase in tissue is due to viscoelastic deformation or 'creep'; one-third is true growth tissue that can be used for reconstruction.

A vascular capsule forms within a week. The increased vascularity makes tissue-expanded flaps more reliable and infections less 'critical' than with other foreign bodies.

Common indications include:

- Breast reconstruction. Expanders can be used to expand the skin prior to replacement by a definitive implant. Alternatively, a permanent composite saline/silicone expander, e.g. Becker or McGhan, can be used to avoid additional surgery.
- Scalp lesions, e.g. alopecia and giant naevi.
- Prefabricated flap. Expanders can be placed under planned skin or muscle flaps to increase the amount of tissue that can be harvested, with the added advantage of thinning out the muscle.

Tissue expansion has many advantages:

- It recruits local skin, which provides the best colour, contour and hair match (where important).
- The tissue can be functional with a robust blood supply and intact nerve supply.
- Donor closure potentially leaves a simple linear scar.

However, the procedure is a major undertaking for the patient.

- Multiple operations, usually two per reconstruction (one to insert, one to remove)
- Multiple visits for expansion of prosthesis
- Carrying a 'disfiguring' lump around for weeks.

Contraindications—generally, tissues that will not stretch, e.g. scarred, grafted or irradiated tissue, and some areas that are notoriously difficult to expand, e.g. the back.

There are a variety of expanders:

- Various shapes can be tailored to requirements. Rectangular implants offer the largest increase in surface area per volume expanded (38% vs 25% for round expanders). An approximate rule of thumb is:
  —Area of base of expander should be 2.5× the area of the defect for rectangular/crescentic expanders.
  —Diameter of expander should be 2.5× the width of the defect for round expanders.
- Backing—some have a firm backing and can be used for areas such as the eyelid, to protect the underlying soft tissues from compression.
- Filling ports may be integral or distant. Distant ports can be internal or exteriorized, which is particularly useful for children.

Incisions:

- radial—reduces tension, less risk of dehiscence, fewer complications
- tangential—parallel and smaller scar, but increased tension means a longer wait before starting.

The pocket needs to be sufficiently large, otherwise the efficiency of expansion is reduced.

Expansion regime

- Individual regimes vary, but typically, expansion commences 1–2 weeks after insertion and the patient returns at approximately weekly intervals for repeated expansion until the final desired volume is reached. In breast reconstruction, over-expansion is followed by partial deflation to recreate ptosis.
- Rapid expansion—patient returns for expansion every 2–3 days. The volume injected is guided by the patient's level of comfort and the skin condition.
- Intraoperative expansion is described but is generally not regarded as being that effective, or only as effective as undermining tissue without providing additional tissue.

Complications—a rate of 5–7% overall is typically quoted, with a higher risk in:

- children, especially the very young, those with burns or prior expansion or tissue loss
- lower limb—50% infection rate.

Common complications:

- Haematoma/seroma
- Implant rupture/migration/extrusion
- Wound dehiscence, which may be due to aggressive over-expansion or poor placement of the incision
- Infection. Due to the good blood supply, infected expanders may still settle with antibiotics and allow completion of the procedure
- Skin necrosis
- Atrophy of neighbouring tissues, especially in young children where underlying bones can be deformed; however, the problem is generally reversible within months.

Further reading

Hudson D, Grob M. Optimising results with tissue expansion: 10 simple rules for successful tissue expander insertion. *Burns* 2005; **31:**1–4.

Related topic of interest

- Breast reconstruction.

Ultraviolet light

The dangers of ultraviolet light in terms of carcinogenesis are well known. It is also responsible for 'general' sun damage to skin, causing premature 'aging' such as wrinkling and pigmentation.

Increased sun exposure has followed the move to hotter climates for holiday destinations or for permanent relocation, and consequently there is an increased cancer risk for fair-skinned Caucasians living in sunny places such as South Africa or Australia. It is estimated that one in two Australians will have non-melanoma skin cancer in their lifetime. Public education is important; **a tan is not healthy**—it represents damage.

The ultraviolet light in sunlight can be classified according to the wavelength:

- Ultraviolet A (UVA) is responsible for 95% of the ultraviolet radiation that reaches our skin. The relatively long wavelength (315–400 nm) compared to ultraviolet B means that it has greater penetration and has the potential to alter the deeper subcutaneous tissues. It tends to cause tanning without much burning.
- Ultraviolet B (UVB) (290–315 nm) is primarily responsible for sunburns and carcinogenesis, which may be related to it effects on immune function. The strongest association is with basal cell carcinomas (BCCs). Eye damage by UVB may lead to cataracts. With depletion of the stratospheric ozone layer, exposure will continue to increase.
- Ultraviolet C (UVC) (200–290 nm) is completely absorbed by ozone and thus is not a cancer risk under normal circumstances.

There is an interaction with:

- **skin type** and complexion of the patient—Fitzpatrick phototypes (1975), as shown in Table 1
- **gender**—different areas are exposed due to different clothing and occupational exposure
- **Genetics:**
  —Xeroderma pigmentosa is an autosomal recessive defect of DNA repair associated with increased risk of skin cancer.

Table 1 Characteristics of the Fitzpatrick phototypes.

Fitzpatrick phototype	Colour of skin	Ultraviolet sensitivity	Reaction to sunlight
I	Extremely fair	Extreme	Always burns, never tans
II	Fair	Very sensitive	Always burns, sometimes tans
III	Medium	Sensitive	Sometimes burns, gradually tans
IV	Olive	Moderate	Occasionally burns, tans well
V	Brown	Minimal	Never burns, tans to dark brown
VI	Black	Insensitive	Never burns, deeply tans

—Albinism is caused by a genetic defect in the tyrosinase enzyme that prevents the production of melanin. It affects both sexes and all races equally; sufferers have an increased risk of BCCs and squamous cell carcinomas, but only rarely have melanomas.

Sunblocks

Conventional sunblocks block UVB far more than they block UVA. Recent studies show that sunblocks may not be as effective as originally thought and that they may encourage greater overall exposure as they instil a false sense of security and thus lead to an increased cancer risk. However, properly used, sunblocks still represent useful protection against the sun, although being 'sun smart' is of greatest importance. As half of a person's lifetime exposure to ultraviolet light occurs before they are 18 years of age; particular care needs to be taken with children.

* Minimize exposure at midday (10 am–2 pm)
* Wear tight-weave clothing, hats and sunglasses
* Avoid using sunbeds.

Sunblocks are usually classified according to their properties:

* **Chemical** or absorptive types. The commonest is para-amino-benzoic acid (PABA) and it is considered to be the best, but it does irritate the skin and stain clothing. Alternatives include PABA esters (padimate O) or cinnamates. Benzophenones are newer chemicals that block both UVA and UVB.
* **Physical** or reflective types, e.g. zinc oxide and titanium oxide. They need to be rubbed in.

Substantivity is a measure of a sunblock's resistance to sweat, water and exercise.

Sunblocks need to be used properly to be effective: they should be applied 30 min before exposure and in good quantity and replenished every 2 h at least. They will only give you protection for a finite time based on your normal tanning/burning time multiplied by the SPF. Thus if you normally burn in half an hour and you use an SPF 15 sunblock (which will block out 95% of the UVB), you can stay out in the sun for $15 \times 30 = 450$ min (7 h 30 min) before you burn. Reapplying more sunblock after this will not give you any more time in the sun.

Further reading

Stanton WR, Janda M, Baade PD, Anderson P. Primary prevention of skin cancer: a review of sun protection in Australia and internationally. *Health Promot Int* 2004; **19:**369–78.

Related topics of interest

* Basal cell carcinoma
* Melanoma
* Squamous cell carcinomas.

Vacuum wound closure

Vacuum wound closure is also known as negative pressure wound therapy (NPWT) and commercially as VAC (vacuum-assisted closure, Kinetic Concepts, Inc.). The concept is that the application of negative, or sub-atmospheric, pressure to selected wounds will speed up their healing and it has been in clinical use since 1993.

The exact mechanism of action is unclear, but there are many theories:

- negative pressure reduces stagnant oedema from the interstitial space. This fluid contains debris, inflammatory mediators and osmotically active substances that would be deleterious to healing
- increases blood flow, which improves oxygen and nutrient delivery
- reduction of bacterial count
- deformational stress increases protein and matrix synthesis and the rate of angiogenesis and formation of granulation tissue
- direct mechanical suction effect that encourages wound contraction similar to a tissue expander effect.

In principle, it is rather simple: a sponge is placed in the wound, covered with an occlusive dressing and connected by tubing to a suction system. The sponge needs to be of a certain porosity and texture to ensure even transmission of the vacuum to the whole wound. More practical control with fewer safety issues is possible with a proprietary system using specific sponges and a machine providing closed-loop controlled programmable suction; this was introduced to the US market in 1995. A portable battery unit is available for ambulatory patients with smaller wounds.

Method

- The wound must be thoroughly debrided to remove any gross necrotic tissue and to open up any tracks/fistulae.
- The wound is covered with a sponge dressing of the same size or slightly smaller. The sponge should not overlie intact skin to avoid maceration.
  - Two types of sponge are offered for their different properties: a black polyurethane sponge is said to encourage granulation tissue formation, whereas a white polyvinyl sponge is more suited to fragile tissues.
  - Applying a non-adherent dressing at the base of the wound may prevent ingrowth of granulation tissue into the sponge, which would make removal painful and bloody.
- Non-collapsible suction tubing is inserted into the sponge and connected up.
- The sponge is covered with an adhesive occlusive dressing with an overlap of 2.5–5 cm. The surrounding skin may be prepared with a hydrocolloid dressing as a base for the adhesive sheet. This is particularly useful for difficult, irregular or moist areas such as the perineum.
- The dressing is changed every 48 h, except when used for skin grafts (4 days).

Pressure

Seminal experiments in animals suggested that intermittent suction (5 min on, 2 min off) is the most effective modality, particularly for encouraging granulation tissue formation. The reasons for this are unclear, but it may be that either the microcirculation or cellular response 'shuts off' with continued stimulation. However, clinicians tend to favour continuous suction because it is less painful and therefore better tolerated.

- Intermittent mode suction is not suitable for heavily exudative wounds because the exudate collecting in the 'off' period may reduce the seal.
- Intermittent suction requires a machine to control the cycling.

Lower pressures 50–75 mmHg may be used for skin grafts or venous ulcers; otherwise, continuous pressure of 125 mmHg is used in the majority of cases.

Problems

- Suction can be painful, particularly with venous ulcers. It may require analgesia; topical local anaesthetic can be applied on the wound or injected through the tubing. One can start at a lower pressure and titrate upward; if the pain is uncontrollable, the treatment may need to be stopped.
- Excessive fluid loss may cause electrolyte or fluid disturbance in large exuding wounds.
- Over-granulation into the sponge may lead to bleeding when the dressing is removed.

Contraindications

- The strongest contraindication is of tumour in the wound; theoretically the increase in blood flow may encourage tumour growth and possibly facilitate movement of malignant cells across tissue planes
- Excessive necrotic tissue or untreated osteomyelitis
- Fistulae may cause large fluid losses though in selected cases vacuum therapy has been used to *close* fistulae.

Other relative contraindications include: arterial disease, heavily infected wounds and patients with bleeding or those on anticoagulants.

Vacuum wound closure can be applied to a wide variety of wounds; there are numerous case reports/studies in the literature. It has been used in venous and diabetic ulcers, pressure sores, and surgical wounds such as sternotomy wounds. In addition, its use in flaps, flap donor sites and split skin graft fixation, particularly on borderline recipient sites, has been described. Its effectiveness seems well established but there is a lack of randomized data comparing it to standard methods. One common concern is that the cost makes clinicians reluctant to use it, although some studies compare it favourably to other treatments in terms of overall cost. Introduction of a wider role for this treatment depends on increased awareness as well as establishing its efficacy in robust randomized controlled trials and demonstrating its cost-effectiveness.

Further reading

Evans D, Land L. Topical negative pressure for treating chronic wounds: a systematic review. *Brit J Plast Surg* 2001: **54**:238–42.

Vascular anomalies

It is vitally important to identify vascular lesions correctly because they have very different clinical behaviours, particularly in their response to surgery. In addition, using consistent and correct nomenclature is vital for meaningful discussion: too often, due to inadequate appreciation of the differences, the terms 'haemangioma', 'vascular malformation' and 'vascular anomalies' are all used interchangeably, leading to confusion when discussing cases, particularly between specialties, and difficulty in comparing studies objectively.

Mulliken and Glowacki studied the cellular components and flow characteristics of the different lesions, providing a framework with standardized definitions that went a long way to improve the general understanding of these lesions:

- Haemangiomas
- Vascular malformations.

The clinical behaviour of these lesions is very different.

Diagnosis is primarily clinical through a thorough history and examination.

MRI is the gold standard investigation but requires a knowledgeable radiologist to interpret them correctly. Biopsy is generally not required as diagnosis is almost always made by history and examination.

Haemangiomas

These are the commonest tumours of infancy (median appearance is at 2 weeks of age) in Caucasians with an increased incidence in the premature. Most cases are sporadic and the cause is unknown. The majority (60%) are found in the head and neck. Females are three times more likely to be affected. The gross appearance is variable: with little overlying tissue, the lesion may appear bright red, ('strawberry naevus') but deeper lesions have a bluish colour ('cavernous haemangioma'). Histology shows hyperplastic endothelium with increased mast cell numbers and rapid endothelial cell turnover.

- **Herald patch** precedes the haemangioma
- **Proliferative phase**, typically occurs during the first 6 months to 2 years
- **Involutional phase**. The general rule of thumb is that 50% of cases will involute by age 5, 70% by age 7 and 90% by age 9. One-third will have a residual grey patch of fibrofatty tissue, which is more likely if involution occurred late. Lesions on the lip and oral cavity are less likely to involute quickly.

As most haemangiomas do involute, the usual treatment is conservative and this is satisfactory in most cases, except for complicated lesions. On average, less than 20% require treatment.

- Bleeding is rarer than might be expected. The Kasabach–Merritt phenomenon is disseminated intravascular coagulopathy; it is frequently mentioned but is very uncommon among the simple haemangiomas (but platelet trapping may lead to a local consumptive coagulopathy in larger lesions).

- Ulceration can be painful and may lead to increased scarring.
- Obstruction of the visual axis or direct compression of the cornea can cause permanent visual problems in a matter of weeks and thus it requires urgent treatment. A short trial of high-dose steroids may be worthwhile before surgery.
- Airway obstruction. Treatment is usually surgical due to its urgency.

Medical treatment
- Systemic steroids (2 mg/kg/day) may be given in a short course with a reasonable response rate. It only works for proliferating lesions. Intralesional steroid injections have been used by some but it is not in common use.
- Subcutaneous injections of IFN2a are slower acting than steroids but will work in non-responders to steroid. Close monitoring is required during treatment: it can cause haemodynamic compromise and the dreaded complication, spastic diplegia, can occur in 10%.
- OK432 (denatured streptococcal protein) stimulates immunologic action and fibrosis.
- Laser treatment has a limited role due to its limited depth of penetration, but pulsed dye lasers (PDL) may be useful to reduce pain in ulcerated lesions. It may lead to scarring and hypopigmentation.
- Embolization has very limited success, possibly due to the small diameter of the vessels involved.

Vascular malformation

These are errors of development and are therefore present from birth, but may not be clinically evident until later on. They tend to grow in proportion to the rest of the body and without any tendency to involute. The endothelium is ultrastructurally normal.

Vascular malformations are classified according to the speed of blood flow through them and the composition of the vessels (see Table 1).

Low-flow lesions
Capillary malformations are commonly called port wine stains (naevus flammeus) and most typically occur in the trigeminal distribution. It begins as a flat and red/pink patch, but with progressive vessel dilatation, it eventually becomes nodular (cobblestoning) and darker. The condition may occasionally be associated with tissue hypertrophy. Traditional treatment options included tattooing, scarification or camouflage, but these have had little role after the advent of laser treatment. The pulse dye laser (PDL) is a useful treatment, but only 10–20% will show near-complete response; the majority only show a partial response and half may recur.

Table 1 Comparison of low-flow and high-flow malformations.

Low-flow malformations	High-flow malformations
Capillary (port wine stains)	Arterial
Venous	Arteriovenous
Lymphatic	

Venous malformations may not be noticed until later in life as a faint blue patch that becomes a soft non-pulsatile compressible blue mass that swells when dependent. These malformations show a predilection for the lips and tongue. Thrombosis and **phleboliths** are characteristic features on imaging. Treatment options include sclerotherapy (alcohol or sodium tetradecyl sulphate) or surgical resection (may have better results with prior sclerosing therapy).

Lymphatic malformations are usually subdivided on the basis of the size of the component cysts.

- Microcystic—commonly called lymphangiomas and tend to be diffuse lesions that cross tissue planes
- Macrocystic—commonly referred to as cystic hygromas. These are more localized and tend to respect tissue planes, making them easier to shell out. They commonly occur in the neck.

Lymphatic malformations do not tend to involute and may increase suddenly if there is infection or bleeding. Treatment options include cautery, radiotherapy and sclerosants, e.g. OK432 or alcohol; these tend to be less effective for microcystic disease. There is a tendency for the lesion to recur if not completely excised. Wound infection and delayed healing is not uncommon.

High-flow lesions

Arterial and arteriovenous malformations are often discussed together. They tend to present later in infancy as a pulsatile lump and enlarge and darken around puberty. They may become painful, ulcerate or bleed and in advanced cases the high-flow can cause high-output heart failure.

Schlobinger staging (1990):

1. Quiescent—blue skin patch
2. Expansion—mass with thrill/bruit
3. Destruction—mass with bleeding/ulceration/pain
4. Decompression—above with heart failure.

In general, treatment is aimed at stage 3 and 4 lesions, and the value of earlier treatment is unclear. Vascular malformations tend to be more difficult to treat compared with haemangomias.

- Simple embolization or ligation of proximal feeding vessels increases the collateral supply and the lesion eventually recurs particularly for high-flow lesions; consequently, this form of treatment is not recommended.
- Arterial lesions need to be excised completely, otherwise recurrence is almost inevitable; completeness of excision may be determined from frozen sections or the pattern of bleeding. Intraoperative bleeding may be profuse; hypotensive anaesthesia, quilting sutures or coagulative aids such as argon plasma may be used.
- In order to reduce bleeding, embolization can be performed 24–72 h prior to surgery.

Syndromic lesions

- **Klippel–Trenaunay–Weber**—an extremity (95% lower limb) port wine stain is associated with a venous/lymphatic or mixed malformation. There may be bony and soft tissue enlargement of the limb. Abnormal lateral leg veins may be present but they should not be ligated as they may represent the only venous drainage for the limb.

- **Osler–Weber–Rendu** (hereditary haemorrhagic telangectasia) is an autosomal dominant condition in which small bright-red arteriovenous malformations are found in perioral skin and mucous membranes.
- In **Sturge–Weber** syndrome, a port wine stain found in the ophthalmic and maxillary areas may be associated with intracranial vascular malformations (leptomeningeal angiomatosis). There may be epilepsy, mental retardation and eye disease such as congenital glaucoma. Dermal staining may involve extremities and trunk, but tissue overgrowth is rare.

Further reading

Muliken JB. Cutaneous vascular anomalies. In: McCarthy JG (ed.). *Plastic Surgery*. Philadelphia: WB Saunders, 1990; 3191–274.

Zygomatic fractures

The typical patient is a young (20–30 years of age) male (80%) involved in an altercation or road traffic accident. The classic 'tripod' fracture actually has four components.

- Zygomatic bone at the zygomaticofrontal (ZF) suture. This is the strongest part of the 'tripod' and if fractured should prompt the active exclusion of other fractures
- Temporal bone alone the zygomatic arch 1.5 cm posterior to the zygomaticotemporal (ZT) suture
- Zygomaticomaxillary buttress in the orbital margin/floor and anterior wall of the maxillary sinus
- Greater wing of the sphenoid in the lateral orbit.

A quarter of patients with zygomatic fractures will have other additional facial fractures.

Assessment

The assessment of a trauma patient always begins with 'ABC': securing the airway with cervical spine control, ensuring breathing and maintaining circulation. Many of these patients will have multiple trauma and serious concomitant injuries need to be excluded as a priority.

- Palpate the bony margins: there may be flattering of malar prominence with a bony step along the infraorbital margin (lateral portion is inferiorly displaced). The masseter can pull the fragment in complex ways—typically medial, inferior and posterior
- Soft tissue bruising and swelling
- Functional
  —An ophthalmic consultation is important as 5% have an associated significant eye injury, and this increases to 20–40% if there is an orbital floor fracture:
    —diplopia (30%) is commonly due to limitation of upward gaze from entrapment of the inferior rectus or contusion. The confirmation of entrapment can be assessed by the forced duction test, which is best done under a general anaesthetic
    —decreased visual acuity may be due to retinal detachment
    —enophthalmos. True globe compression is uncommon
    —subconjunctival haematoma with no posterior limit
    —subcutaneous emphysema.
  —Mouth opening. Trismus may be due to a depressed zygomatic arch fracture impeding movement of the coronoid process underneath it or due to masseter spasm.
  —There may be paraesthesia in the infraorbital nerve territory.

Classification

The commonest system is the Knight and North classification, which subdivides fractures on the basis of their displacement and depression.

Diagnosis

- History and examination is the mainstay of clinical fracture diagnosis.
- Plain radiographs generally offer poor views of the zygoma due to temporal bone shadows.
  —Submentovertex (SMV) view can show the zygomatic arches
  —Waters (37° occipitomental) view for the zygomatic arches and maxillary sinus
  —PA and lateral.
- Fine-cut CT (coronal and axial) is useful for preoperative assessment of the injury, particularly of the orbital wall.

Management

One needs to consider:

- functional problems, e.g. jaw opening
- cosmetic issues, e.g. asymmetry.

Conservative treatment (analgesia, nursing head up, soft diet and no nose blowing) is a suitable option for stable and undisplaced fractures with no functional problems.

Closed reduction may be suitable for a very selective set of patients but is an uncommon option now.

Gillies lift for a depressed zygomatic arch fracture. Care needs to be taken to avoid causing a secondary fracture of the temporal bone by using the bone as a pivot. An alternative is direct percutaneous lift with a clip or hook. Fixation is usually unnecessary in isolated arch fracture but depends on the stability after elevation.

Open reduction and internal fixation is the mainstay of modern treatment of tripod fractures; 80–95% of fractures require open reduction. The surgical principles (as with all fractures) are:

- adequate exposure
- precise reduction
- accurate stabilization.

Some advocate that at least two fractures should be plated; Davidson compared fixation techniques and found stable fixation with plating of the ZF suture and one other; single-site fixation is acceptable in certain situations. Fractures may be accessed by:

- ZF suture via lateral brow incision
- infraorbital rim via subciliary or transconjunctival lower eyelid incision. The eyelid incision offers easy access but is usually avoided because of obvious scarring and the risk of lower lid oedema, even though the risk of other lower lid abnormalities is minimal
- maxilla via upper buccal sulcus incisions.

Wires are an alternative to miniplates (they are cheap and easy to use) but require more exposure. Resorbable plates (3–12 months) are sometimes recommended for children but have a higher profile and require tapping.

Timing of surgery

A zygomatic fracture is not an emergency and if surgery cannot be performed before oedema sets in, then it can be safely postponed and performed as soon as practical before 2–3 weeks. Late surgery (weeks) is hindered by the healed fracture/callus and soft tissue fibrosis.

Complications of surgery

- Nerve injury to infraorbital occurs in up to 20% of patients
- Eye injury
  —persistent diplopia
  —blindness (0.3%) is thankfully rare. It may be due to bone fragments or oedema impinging on the optic nerve. Orbital exploration in the presence of globe rupture or hyphaema can exacerbate injury, underlining the importance of eye consultation.
- Late plate complications such as mechanical failure.

Further reading

Zingg M, Laedrach K, Chen J et al. Classification and treatment of zygomatic fracture: a review of 1025 cases. *J Oral Maxillofac Surg* 1992; **50:**778–90.

Index

abbreviations xi–xii
abdominoplasty 1–2
acids, chemical burns 34
actinic keratosis (solar keratosis) 150
adenoid cystic carcinomas 147
adenolymphomas (Warthin's tumour) 147
alkali, chemical burns 34
'AMPLE' history 4
anaesthetic complications 43–4
anaesthetics, local 113–16
  action 114
  commonly used 113–14
  EMLA (eutectic mixture of local
    anaesthetics) 116
  topical anaesthetics 116
  types 114–16
anatomy, facial 65–8
Apert's syndrome, craniosynostosis 49–51
arrhythmias, electrical burns 59

basal cell carcinoma (BCC) 9–11
botulinum toxin 12–14
Bowens disease 150–1
breast augmentation 15–18
  breast feeding 18
  complications 16–17
  implant types 15
  mammography 18
  placement 15–16
  safety 17–18
breast reconstruction 19–22
  free flaps 20–1
  immediate/delayed 19–20
  implant types 19–20
  pedicled flaps 20
breast reduction 23–5
  alternatives to surgery 24–5
  complications 24
  oncology 25
  pedicles 23–4
  postoperative care 24
  techniques 23–4
burn dressings 26–9
  antimicrobials 28
  basic 27
  definitive 27
  first aid 26
  MRSA 26
  occlusive 27–8
  properties 26
  regimes 29
  SSD 28

TSS 26
  types 27–9
burn surgery 30–2
  early 30
  meshing 31–2
  SSG 31
  wound closure 31–2
burns, acute 3–8
  area 6–7
  assessment 5–7
  decompression 7
  features 6
  first aid 3–4
  infection 8
  inhalation injury 4–5
  Jackson's burn model 3
  nutrition 8
  pain relief 8
  resuscitation 7
  types 3
burns, chemical 33–5
  acids 34
  alkali 34
  extravasation injuries 35
  first aid 33
  surgery 34–5
burns, electrical 58–60
  compartment syndrome 58
  first aid 59
  management 59–60
burns, paediatric 142–5
  depth 142
  first aid 142
  long-term effects 143–4
  NAI 144
  resuscitation 143
  surface area 142–3
  TSS 144

cancer see carcinoma
capillary malformations 182–3
carcinoma
  actinic keratosis (solar keratosis) 150
  adenoid cystic carcinomas 147
  BCC 9–11
  Bowens disease 150–1
  erythroplakia 150
  leukoplakia 150
  lymphomas 147
  melanoma 121–5
  mucoepidermoid carcinomas 147
  neck dissection 129–33

oral cancer 138–41
    parotid gland tumours 146–9
    premalignant lesions 150–1
    see also squamous cell carcinomas
CFNG *see* cross-facial nerve grafting
chemical burns 33–5
chromophores, lasers 105
cleft lip 36–8
    Millard rotation-advancement 37
    postoperative care 37–8
    presurgical orthopaedics 38
    Skoog 37
    surgical techniques 37
    Tennison–Randall 37
    timing 36
    treatment 36–7
cleft palate 39–42
    classification 39
    embryology 39
    operative repair 41
    problems 39–40
    surgical techniques 40–1
    timing 40
    Veau–Kilner–Wardill technique 40
    Von Lagenbeck technique 40
    VPI 41
clostridial myonecrosis 135
compartment syndrome, electrical burns 58
complications 43–8
    anaesthetic 43–4
    haematoma 45
    haemorrhage 45
    hypoxia 46–7
    laser 47
    pyrexia 46
    smoking 43
    wound infection 44–5
consent, informed 98–9
craniosynostosis 49–51
    Apert's syndrome 49–51
    Crouzon's syndrome 49
cross-facial nerve grafting (CFNG), facial
        reanimation 73
Crouzon's syndrome, craniosynostosis 49

DD *see* Dupuytren's disease
decompression, acute burns 7
distal interphalangeal joint (DIPJ), extensor
        tendon injuries 62–3
dressings
    pressure sores 153
    see also burn dressings
Dupuytren's disease (DD) 52–4
    risk factors 52–3
    staging 53
    treatment 53–4

ear, facial anatomy 67
ear reconstruction 55–7
    microtia 55
    prostheses 57
    timing 56–7
ears, prominent 155–7
    complications 156–7
    management 155
    non-surgical treatment 155
    postoperative care 156
    surgery 155–6
electrical burns 58–60
EM *see* erythema multiforme
EMLA (eutectic mixture of local
        anaesthetics) 116
erythema multiforme (EM) *see*
        Stevens–Johnson syndrome
erythroplakia 150
express consent 98
extensor tendon injuries 61–4
    anatomy 61
    complications 63–4
    distal interphalangeal joint (DIPJ) 62–3
    management 61–2
    metacarpophalangeal joint (MCPJ) 63
    proximal interphalangeal joint (PIPJ) 63
    rehabilitation 63
extravasation injuries, chemical burns 35
eye, facial anatomy 65

facial anatomy 65–8
    ear 67
    eye 65
    lip 66
    nose 68
facial hypoplasia 92–4
    hemifacial atrophy of Romberg 93
    hemifacial microsomia 92–3
    TCS 92
facial lacerations 69–71
    deeper lacerations 69–70
    nerves 70–1
    skin lacerations 69
facial reanimation 72–4
    CFNG 73
    muscle restoration 73–4
    nerve crossovers 73
    nerve restoration 72–3
fine needle aspiration cytology (FNAC),
        parotid gland tumours 148
first aid
    acute burns 3–4
    burn dressings 26
    chemical burns 33
    electrical burns 59
    paediatric burns 142

Fitzpatrick phototypes, ultraviolet light 177
fleur-de-lis-shaped incision 1
flexor tendon injuries 75–81
   complications 81
   digital flexor sheath 75
   examination 77–8
   healing mechanism 76–7
   management 77
   nutrition 75–6
   postoperative care 80–1
   surgery 78–9
FNAC *see* fine needle aspiration cytology
fractures
   mandibular 82–5
   zygomatic 185–7

grafts, skin *see* skin grafts
greater trochanter, pressure sores 154
gynaecomastia 86–8

haemangiomas 181–2
haematoma, complications 45
haemorrhage, complications 45
hair removal 89–91
   laser 90–1
   methods 89–90
   temporary reduction of hair 90
hemifacial atrophy of Romberg, facial
     hypoplasia 93
hemifacial microsomia, facial hypoplasia 92–3
hypertrophic scarring 100–2
hypoplastic facial conditions *see* facial
     hypoplasia
hypospadias 95–7
   assessment 95–6
   complications 97
   surgery 96–7
hypoxia, complications 46–7

IMF *see* intermaxillary fixation
implant types
   breast augmentation 15
   breast reconstruction 19–20
implied consent 98
infection, acute burns 8
informed consent 98–9
inhalation injury, acute burns 4–5
intermaxillary fixation (IMF), mandibular
     fractures 84–5
ischial sores, pressure sores 154

Jackson's burn model 3

KA *see* keratoacanthoma
keloids 100–2
keratoacanthoma (KA) 164

Klippel–Trenaunay–Weber, vascular anomaly
   183–4

lacerations, facial 69–71
Laser Doppler imaging (LDI), acute burns 5
lasers
   applications 104–5
   chromophores 105
   CO_2 laser 104
   complications 47
   hair removal 90–1
   hypertrophic scarring 102
   keloids 102
   principles 103–6
   Q-switched (QS) 172–4
   selectivity 105
   tattoo removal 172–4
LDI *see* Laser Doppler imaging
leg ulcers 107–9
   appearance 108
   investigations 107
   management 107–9
   surgery 109
   treatment 107–9
   venous ulcers 107
leukoplakia 150
lip, facial anatomy 66
liposuction 1, 110–12
   complications 112
   fluid infiltration 110–11
   techniques 110–11
   types 110–11
local anaesthetics *see* anaesthetics, local
lymphatic malformations 183
lymphoedema 117–20
   differential diagnosis 117–18
   investigations 118
   management 118–20
   physiotherapy 119
   surgery 119–20
lymphomas 147

mammography, breast augmentation 18
mandibular fractures 82–5
   assessment 83
   complications 85
   condylar fractures 85
   favourable/unfavourable 82
   imaging 83–4
   IMF 84–5
   treatment 84
melanoma 121–5
   historical subtypes 121–2
   investigations 123–4
   lymph nodes management 124
   prognostic factors 122–3

risk factors 121
signs 122
staging 123
meshing
  burn surgery 31–2
  skin grafts 163
metacarpophalangeal joint (MCPJ), extensor
    tendon injuries 63
microsurgery and tissue transfer 126–8
  postoperative management 126–7
  potential problems 127–8
microtia, ear reconstruction 55
Millard rotation-advancement, cleft lip 37
Mohs' micrographic surgery (MMS),
    BCC 10
mouth, oral cancer 138–41
MRSA, burn dressings 26
mucoepidermoid carcinomas 147
muscle restoration, facial reanimation 73–4

NAI *see* non-accidental injury
neck dissection 129–33
  assessment 129
  complications 132
  lymph nodes classification 130
  neck nodes levels 129
  RND 130–1
  skin incisions 132–3
  surgical management 129–32
necrotizing fasciitis (NF) 134–5
  clostridial myonecrosis 135
  investigations 135
  polymicrobial 134
  streptococcal 134–5
  treatment 135
  types 134–5
nerve crossovers, facial reanimation 73
nerve restoration, facial reanimation 72–3
nerves, facial lacerations 70–1
neurofibromatosis 136–7
NF *see* necrotizing fasciitis
non-accidental injury (NAI), paediatric burns
  144
nose
  facial anatomy 68
  see also rhinoplasty
nutrition
  acute burns 8
  flexor tendon injuries 75–6

oncology, breast reduction 25
oral cancer 138–41
  assessment 138–9
  treatment 139–41
Osler–Weber–Rendu, vascular anomaly
  184

paediatric burns 142–5
pain relief, acute burns 8
parotid gland tumours 146–9
  adenoid cystic carcinomas 147
  adenolymphomas (Warthin's tumour) 147
  benign 146–7
  FNAC 148
  investigations 148–9
  lymphomas 147
  malignant 147
  mucoepidermoid carcinomas 147
  PSAs 146
  superficial parotidectomy 148–9
physiotherapy, lymphoedema 119
pleiomorphic salivary adenomas (PSAs) 146
plication of the recti 1
polymicrobial necrotizing fasciitis 134
premalignant lesions 150–1
pressure sores 152–4
  causes 152
  management 153–4
prostheses, ear reconstruction 57
proximal interphalangeal joint (PIPJ),
    extensor tendon injuries 63
PSAs *see* pleiomorphic salivary adenomas
pyrexia, complications 46

Q-switched (QS) lasers 172–4

radical neck dissection (RND), neck
    dissection 130–1
radiotherapy, hypertrophic scarring/keloids
    102
von Recklinghausen's disease 136–7
resuscitation
  acute burns 7
  paediatric burns 143
  see also first aid
rhinoplasty 158–60
  complications 160
  examination 158
  history 158
  postoperative care 160
  surgery 159–60
rhytides (wrinkles) 12–14
RND *see* radical neck dissection
rodent ulcer 9–11

sacral sores, pressure sores 154
SAL *see* suction-assisted liposuction
scarring, hypertrophic 100–2
SCC *see* squamous cell carcinomas
silicone breast implants 15–18
silver sulphadiazine (SSD), burn dressings
  28
SJS *see* Stevens–Johnson syndrome

skin grafts 161–3
  composite 163
  meshing 163
  thickness 162
  see also tissue expansion; tissue transfer and
    microsurgery
Skoog, cleft lip 37
smoking, complications 43
solar keratosis (actinic keratosis) 150
split-thickness skin grafts (SSG), burn surgery
  31
squamous cell carcinomas (SCC) 164–5
  KA 164
  management 164–5
  oral cancer 138–41
  premalignant lesions 150–1
  risk factors 164
  treatment 165
SSD *see* silver sulphadiazine
SSG *see* split-thickness skin grafts
Stevens–Johnson syndrome (SJS) 166–8
streptococcal necrotizing fasciitis 134–5

Sturge–Weber syndrome 184
suction-assisted liposuction (SAL) 1
sunblocks, ultraviolet light 178
surgery, chemical burns 34–5
suturing 169–71
  alternatives to excision 171
  alternatives to sutures 171
  classification 170
  principles 169
  removing sutures 170–1
  types of stitching 169

tattoo removal 172–4
  complications 173–4
  lasers 172–4
  treatment options 172–3
TCS *see* Treacher–Collins syndrome
TEN *see* toxic epidermal necrolysis
tendons *see* extensor tendon injuries; flexor
  tendon injuries
Tennison–Randall, cleft lip 37
tissue expansion 175–6